Once I was Old
Now I am Young at 81
True Story

There is no one else but you –
without you there is nothing.

Roger L. Mathis N.C.C.H.T.

ISBN: 978-0-9815151-0-6
Library of Congress Control Number:

Edited by Jamie Eagle
Cover Design by High Level Studios
Book layout and design by Just Ink courtesy of High Level Studios
www.highlevelstudios.com

This book is printed on acid-free paper

TABLE OF CONTENTS

INTRODUCTION

Please allow me to introduce myself. My name is Roger L. Mathis, NCCHT. I was born in September 1926 in St. Louis, Missouri. I have studied at three universities in St. Louis and am proud to have served my country in World War II from 1943 to 1946. My duties were in the air group on the *USS Hornet* Aircraft Carrier CV-12. I participated in the invasion of both Iwo Jima and Okinawa, in the Battle of Leyte and Samara, in the Philippines Liberation, and in addition, was given the presidential unit citation from the Secretary of the Navy. I have studied and maintained certificates in homeopathic medicine, nutritional counseling, and certified hypnotherapy for both adults and pediatrics. I am the proud father of six beautiful children—three boys and three girls. They look at me, their father, as their doctor of health. I am currently in my eighties and still run every day. I've conquered fourteen marathons. I look like and act as a man who is thirty-five years younger.

Are you ready to learn more about me?

I have a multivitamin made up of my own personal formula, which is called Ad-ditions. It has been on the market for sixteen years. Ad-ditions is sold in two of the large grocery chains in Missouri and Indiana. My product is designed to improve energy and supplement the essential vitamins and minerals needed to obtain optimal health.

Are you ready to learn more about me?

I have lectured for years in the eastern part of the United States about anti-aging, while also selling the Ad-ditions multivitamin.

This book contains deep, provocative subject matter with which I don't believe many people have been confronted. I chose to title my book *Once I Was Old, Now I Am Young At 81* mainly because it is true, and I'll explain as I go on.

Throughout my entire life, I always thought that there was someone who was going to be around no matter what happened. I looked at true love as being a part of it all, but over time, I realized love was not the whole answer. What I have observed in my lifetime is that most people who live together, such as family, mothers, fathers, and children, all depend on someone else to help them and take care of them, or at least give them suggestions.

I never was so wrong in all my life.

In the past, I had a lot going on in my life, and I didn't have the intellect at the time to realize that there was no one else around but me. I can give you a number of examples, but I guess the one that started it all was when I married my children's mother. After twenty-three years of marriage, I was confronted with getting a divorce. The divorce was, in all probability, no one's fault because I don't believe anymore that a divorce can be the fault of one person. It's a case where someone is dependant upon another, and the spouse (or whoever may be involved) is not there at the time in which the other needs them the most. At certain times, the relationship breaks down because there is a lack of communication or understanding. It is frightening when you are confronted with this situation. In a divorce, it is troubling to realize the complications involved with the departed spouse, which include the children, relatives, friends, and all of the relationships that you have developed over a number of years.

People only think about themselves in any given situation. No matter how severe or traumatic, most people will eventually disregard your importance as time goes by. You can devote years to caring for someone, but over a period of time, it becomes emotional and aggravating. It gets to a point where some think they want a better life. They will not and cannot do it anymore. This is the point that I am trying to reiterate to my readers. If you think for one moment there's anyone out there, regardless of how close they may be to you at this present moment, who will always be there for you, I believe that you should forget this. You only have yourself and that is the reason I am writing this book and providing all of the detailed information about alternatives to medications.

You should try to make your life better. It is not good enough trying to find someone out there who's going to love you and whom you can depend on. Some day when you are disabled, sick, or whatever it may be, when you are in a situation where it's an inconvenience for someone else, you can rest assured that this person will no longer be your friend or have anything to do with you anymore. I am still relating to my divorce with my children's mother. With all due respect to everybody that was involved, I had thought they were the greatest people that ever lived. I loved them all; there were no exceptions. I thought I had a great deal of nothing but wonderful relationships.

When I divorced my children's mother after twenty-three

years, it was for another woman. The reason that I made that decision was solely because I was not getting what I wanted out of our marriage: love. Love comes in many different forms and from many different people who have different ways of expressing themselves. I don't believe there's anything on this earth that is more special than a show of love in every capacity. In my particular situation, once the divorce was finalized, every single friend of mine disappeared. There was no one there, not even my children. And at the time, I gave up because of my guilt. I gave up everything that I owned—the house, the cars, the furnishings —everything you can think of. With regard to child support and alimony, no matter who I tried to get assistance from, I was rejected by every single person. Divorce can put an enormous amount of financial burden on an individual. As a result, my self-esteem went down the toilet. If you can imagine for a moment, it seemed like I was living in a world with millions of people, yet there was no out there who wanted to have anything to do with me. I felt like a leper—like I was living in a colony by myself. I entered a deep state of depression, not knowing where to go or what to do.

When I moved out after the first divorce, I lived in an apartment. I found an apartment with no furnishings, including no bed, because I was not allowed to have anything at the time. I had a knock on the door to the apartment one day, and one of my sons came in and asked if he could live with me. He knew I didn't have anything, but he decided he wanted to live with me. So we found a bed and stayed together for a while. He, out of all the people in this world, came to me and wanted to live with me.

This was basically my salvation. My two youngest girls, ages seven and nine, were also extremely instrumental in my salvation.

Their mother was still hurting from the divorce and was hesitant about giving me visitation rights. Nevertheless, my two little girls still wanted to see me, despite what their mother wanted. The love they had for me then is still there and even more powerful today. What's even better is that they project this amount of love to their mother, too. After twenty-five years, I talk to their mother every once in a while. I try to accept and understand her bitterness toward me.

There was extreme hate for me from one of my sons. He punished me by the way he treated me and through his refusal to talk to me for years. That alone tore my heart apart. This went on until he married. Then he realized why certain things happen in life. I'm happy to say that currently we are all talking again. To this day, I have felt I was blessed that he came into my life more so than ever before. He assisted me in a way he didn't realize because he knew deep down that it isn't just one person's fault when there is a divorce. Time has a way of healing all.

After a period of time seeking help from psychologists and psychiatrists, and feeling a sickness that just wouldn't leave, the sickness penetrated my mind. They could never figure out why I felt so terrible. There had to be something wrong. I would like to remind you that when I came out of the military after World War II, I was a basket case. I remember coming out and experiencing a state of depression that you wouldn't believe. I did nothing but cry all of the time. I saw many physicians, psychiatrists, and psychologists. This went on for years. I could never figure out what was wrong, and I kept my depression within me. I cannot blame all the people who were around me. If I would have had enough self-esteem at the time, maybe I would have had a more productive life. I was depressed and had lost everything, but I had to keep going, and I did.

At that time, I started seeking out other methods of treatment. These were vitamins and nutrition, various things which took many years of research to understand. I point this out because my depression went on as long as I let it go on; it was partially my fault. I could find no assistance, and this is what made me strong over a period of time.

I went on to remarry and, because of the lack of interest my chosen mate had with my children, I had to let it go. I married again after about ten years and the same thing happened again. I loved my children more than anything else on this earth. Whether they loved me or not wasn't important; I wasn't going to give up on any of them, regardless of what happened after the divorce. My guilt and my impression of myself was something I had to overcome. One of the main reasons that I am writing this book is because I want to let all the readers know that it was up to me. There was no one out there that would have stayed with me because I didn't want help. I wanted some miracle.

I've always been devoted to God and I prayed heavily about everything that was going on. In fact, I was on the verge of committing suicide. My suicidal tendencies were very dominant. I was trying to find someone to care for me via my relationships with women. Nothing ever worked. No matter what I did, everything seemed to end in failure. I didn't get along with people because of my attitude, obviously, but no matter where I went, the help I was seeking was never there.

When I look back in retrospect, I think about how scary my

suicidal tendencies were. I remember one evening going to bed when I was living in my apartment. I was extremely depressed and very much into prayer at the time. Prayer didn't seem to do much good, but I still prayed continuously even though I had lost my religion after being excommunicated from the Catholic Church when I got a divorce. That night, I took my pistol to bed with me and told God as I knelt by the side of my bed to please give me some help. I prayed that night that if I woke up the next morning and still felt the same way, I was going to kill myself. This was the first miracle that was preformed, in my opinion, by my prayers and devotion to God.

I woke up the next morning and felt like a whole new person. I did not want to kill myself anymore and felt that I was on my way to something, though I didn't know what it was. From that moment on, however, I had nothing but struggles. I continuously had financial problems, but I still never lost my love for my children. It seemed like everywhere I went I was always running into a brick wall, especially because I was carrying guilt. When you constantly carry around guilt, it's like a truckload of cement on your back. You are never going to get anywhere.

After about seven years, I finally decided to go back and try to find another church. I found a church in which I became a little bit active. I finally went up to the front of the church at the end of a service and told the pastor and many others what was going on in my life. They told me that I was carrying an enormous amount of guilt by leaving my children's mother. I knelt down with all of these people and prayed that I would be relieved of my guilt. Fortunately, my troubles seemed to lift enormously after a lot of help and prayers were provided by the people that I met at that church. I knew that I had to keep going and find other means to keep my troubles away.

Here again are the reasons why I am taking the time to give you an idea of what it takes in life. There is no one else but you, and you have to find your own way. If you are in a situation where you have many friends and relationships, you're blessed. But don't ever depend on those to last forever. You have to make them last, and when all is said and done, you will be victorious, just as I am now.

When I was finally able to move on with my life, I became a nutrition counselor and a certified hypnotherapist for both adults and children. I won't bore you with the details of how I came to this point, but I just want to let you know that the fear and guilt that many people carry around during their lifetime is a killer, and it almost killed me. The one thing I did that helped me more than anything was getting up and running every single day. I still do this. I also started developing better relationships with my children. Over a period of time, I acquired the friendship of my two little ones when they were still small.

One of the most interesting things about all of this is that in life, people admire and respect other people for what they are, what they do, and what they have. Unfortunately, I was not wealthy at the time this all happened. I was fairly successful, but I was not a big man at 5'9". I always thought I was an attractive man, and I still do, but one thing that people always admire is a person's success, which is measured by what one has. Unfortunately, if I had been a wealthy man, I do not think my divorce would have been treated the way it was. People often judge others by their stature. I'm convinced that when you're not tall, you don't have all of the ingredients to win the admiration of others. When you have money, everyone wants to be around you. When you have a lot of money, you are able to gather more friends.

Unfortunately, I did not have those assets, and it's a shame because that is what life is all about. It's about how you feel about yourself. I know there have been short people in the world who have been successful in different ways. I can think of a few. Harry Truman was president of the United States, even though he was not a tall man. Hitler was a noted person. I'm sure that he was not without friends. No matter where you look, you will always find that those people with a lot of money get divorced, kill people, and get off easy because they've got the money to buy their way out.

I want to show you that whatever your problem may be, I truly believe you can successfully gain control of it. You need to work at finding what you need, even if you have to pay for it. That was the hardest thing I had to do. I had owed a lot of people money. I was in debt and some people, including a few of my sons, got together and gave me some assistance. I didn't even have a place to live at times. One of my sons actually brought me into his household. I lived with him for a long period of time until I could find other people who were interested in me. I have always been interested in nutrition and I found people out there who wished to help me as time went on. I just never gave up. The only reason I didn't succeed earlier was because I was still having stress that was driving me insane.

This book will show you what I did and what I found that can help you become a better person. This might all sound like doom and gloom, but it's not to be presented that way because I really do believe that there is a light. I am living some of it now at the age of eighty. If you feel like you are not in a successful mode or are depressed and having problems, please seek help, even if it costs money. Because I am a World War II veteran and have been in combat, my mind has been affected. When you can't think straight, things don't work right. You just have to try to keep yourself going, and if you're feeling bad, you must find ways to feel better. God made each of us different. In this life, I don't know what he wants us to learn. The thing I've found is that you have to work hard at life. Life isn't easy, and if you expect it to be easy, that's another tragic mistake you'll make.

Listen to my story, good people, for I believe I have experienced just about everything that life has to offer. Fortunately, even with all the problems I have had, no doctor ever told me that I had anything physically wrong with me. My problems seemed to revolve around my anxiety and stress. I experienced anxiety and panic attacks. I remember having panic attacks and calling people at three or four o'clock in the morning trying to get someone to give me assistance, but there was no one. If you have never had a panic attack, God blessed you. In a panic attack, you completely lose control of yourself and lose all of your reasoning on how to overcome the situation. It is an extremely frightening experience. Like I said before, everybody had removed me from their lives, even my children. They have all come back now, but it took me many years of always loving them to regain what I had. I always knew that I had to do it on my own. Without me, I am nothing.

On my lecturing tours, it was alarming to learn how many adults and children were not taking vitamins or mineral supplements. I was also appalled by their diets, which consisted mostly of fried and fast foods. I interviewed hundreds of adults and teenagers all fixed on junk food. My stance is this: You eat what you want. However, let me eat what is healthy so that I can be rewarded with longevity and be disease-free. Most people, including myself, have learned the hard way. People know when they have eaten a particular food that makes their body react in a negative way. This is because all people, both young and old, have different body chemistries. The learning process comes with time.

This book will hopefully introduce you to many of the strategies that will help you maintain a healthier life. It is being written for the benefit of hundreds and hundreds of people who have continuously questioned how I look so young. My six beautiful children—Roger, Deborah, Mark, Craig, Lisa, and Tina—tell me that if I die before this book is completed, they will kill me. So I'm going to be fighting a losing battle either way.

I have asked myself this question many times: What contribution does any person have to offer the world when one possesses only self-worth and does not care for others?

Throughout my lifetime, I have had times of zero self-worth when I never felt good about anything. I was thinking only of myself and never about those around me. The complaining I did was continuous. It was then that I realized that no one cared about my problems. It was only little old me. This brought me into depression, gave me anxiety, and I suffered from more and more health ailments. I would be ashamed to tell anyone about the many doctors who were being paid immeasurable amounts of my money. Not one of these doctors gave me anything positive to work with. Because I was a World War II veteran who participated in combat in the South Pacific, most of my issues were pinned on that. Many of the medications that I was taking literally put me on the floor or made me bedridden. After being medicated, sometimes I would shake so badly that my body felt like it was coming apart. Many years passed, and I rarely considered any of my days "good" days. If I did, I would question why.

My life was what I considered turmoil. I'd had three marriages and a bankruptcy, but I was still trying to make a living. There were no friends present in my life. I was considering suicide and there was no one to talk to. My children did not understand. However, everything changed that fateful night when I made a pact with God. I felt happier, and I knew it was time to start helping myself.

There were two supports to my survival. One support was that I had been a runner for most of my life. Running was enjoyable and took care of some of the depression and loneliness. It was also a support to me throughout the forthcoming years when the people I met asked my age. They were all astonished by how I looked much younger. In the beginning, and most of the time, this meant nothing to me. However, after this carried on for years, I was affected, which is precisely why this book is being written.

As I mentioned, I was born in September 1926, so I am currently in my eighties. Never in my mind did I think I would live to this age, but I'm still going strong and am told I look forty-five to fifty. Everyone I speak to wants to know my secret, which I am now ready to reveal to those who want to look and feel much younger. Let's talk. Let me inform you, dear readers, that anything worthwhile in life takes time. My brief explanation of some of the tribulations that I experienced in life is to let you know that you can be healthy and look ever-loving younger when you follow these formulas.

For fifty-five years or more, I have researched just about every form of minerals, vitamins, and supplements. These supplements play a significant part of one's body chemistry. I have personally consumed every supplement you will be reading about. I have positive proof that they help prevent many diseases. Each of us have our own feelings and personalities, so therefore these chemicals work differently within each of us and thus seem to change every seven years. When chemicals change, as they most assuredly will, this is a time of learning. You may visit practitioners with your feelings, positive or negative. You alone make the good come into reality. Do not stop looking for that good answer.

There is a saying that I think has a great deal of substance in regards to what we are in life and what we do with our existence. It goes something like this: Is there an existence in life without wanting to help others? I don't think so. In life, there is no other way to have a meaningful existence than to have a desire to live to see other people live and to research everything that there is on earth. I think that everything on earth, regardless of its seeming magnitude or insignificance, is worth researching to find out why it is here. God did not create anything without reason. You need to determine whether things are good or bad. God put some things on this earth that we consider bad, but when you actually research them, you'll find out a different answer. We have so much to learn about life and its existence. Most of all, we must learn how to live longer.

After spending many years researching and looking into the problems of a normal human being, I've found that the question "why" is the one thing in life causing more diseases than anything else on earth. You take pages to describe what is bothering you and why you are suffering from some disease. There are some parts of your life that are not desirable. Perhaps you are crippled or you were born with a disease. Maybe it stems from our relationship with the big unbelievable word: FEAR.

Fear, in my opinion, causes all kinds of diseases. Fear is the worst thing you can have in your life. I'm also pretty sure that almost everyone has a fear of dying—I know I do. I've researched a great deal over the years to figure out why I was feeling at my worst. I visited many doctors. Fear, I finally figured out, is the most relative thing to all that is wrong with us. You can be sick, disabled, crippled, born with certain infirmities—you can have anything. However, you can be a decent, strong, happy, and loving human being when you do not have fear. Fear comes from so many directions. I have been in a fearful state most of my life.

Why does a person begin his life in fear? I think it stems from our parents and our ancestors. You are a product of your environment and upbringing, whatever it may be. That product of the environment comes, in my humble opinion, from fear. I have seen how doctors treat symptoms. They suppress the symptom with some form of a painkiller, which slows you down, numbs your brain, and changes your thought processes. As long as you stay in that same state, for whatever period of time, your fear somewhat subsides. That's why there are so many tranquilizers sold in pharmacies and prescribed by doctors, because they do make you feel better for a short period of time. When you look at prescription drugs and the side effects that they have, maybe it's okay to take them for a while. You can feel better and maybe they boost your immune system to protect you from many of the things that are bothering you.

I have found this out personally. Some of the things that were bothering me during my lifetime were driving me insane. I tried all of the other methods that we just talked about. I tried them and they worked for a while, but then they just stopped. It's just like everything in life—after a period of time you always become immune to something. Take a vitamin, take a drug, take anything, and after a period of time, the effectiveness that comes from the product you're taking will eventually lose its potency because you become immune to it.

I could never figure out why pharmacists and doctors write the same prescriptions for or suggest the same over-the-counter drugs to people who weigh 300 pounds and people who weigh 100 pounds. Heavier people have more fat and more cells, so they've got more of a chance to get to the problem, whatever it may be. Some doctors do take weight into consideration, but for the most part, every doctor will prescribe the same medications regardless of how much you weigh or how tall you are. I find this disturbing only because you see smaller people coming back to doctors to have them weaken or change the prescription because it just hit them too hard. Women and older people have that problem also, especially if they are not exercising or utilizing their brain.

I just want to emphasize how important it is to understand why you are not feeling well. When you are not feeling well, what's the first thing you think about? Maybe I've got something, maybe I'm sick. This is a fear for you. That's all it is. Sometimes you need to accept some of the problems because this is the first and only thing that you can do to start the healing process.

This book will hopefully assist you in your life journey. Life is not easy. In fact, it can be damn hard, especially if your health is not up to par. My experiences will give you the guidelines I wish I would've had earlier on in my life. How much time you wish to devote to good health is entirely up to you. Remember one thing and one thing only: You can't have the life you would like to have without good health. Let my experiences be your shortcut to health and happiness. The following chapters will give you the insight and knowledge you need to achieve the wellbeing you desire.

SECTION 1
THE BODY

DAILY SCHEDULE

People always ask me how I stay looking so young. They ask about my skin and tell me it looks beautiful. These people have been complimenting me for years. Most of my family has told me that I need to elaborate on my methods and explain how to maintain such great health.

I want to tell you about my daily schedule and what I do each and every morning. I have talked to you about the supplements that I take. However, if you're not taking care of your skin, you are making a big mistake! Your skin is the largest organ on your body and conveys many signs of sickness and diseases that may occur. So the treatment of your skin, both internally and externally, is going to affect the way you look, the way you feel, and the quality of your life. What we all strive for is longevity. Longevity has to do with the quality of your life, and if we don't have a good quality of life, we have nothing.

First of all, I'd like to talk about what I do in the mornings. Before I get out of bed, I actually massage my entire body with the fingertips of both hands. I massage for a period of about five to ten minutes and I work on every part of my body. I take my fingertips and massage away from my forehead, over my face, to my eyes, and to my temples. I go into each segment of all the curves, and this also extends to the ears.

Rubbing your ears can actually stimulate circulation to other parts of the body. Do not miss your ears when you are doing your facial massage in the morning. You should rub the top of your ears, the outer part of all the curvatures, along the borderlines of the outer ear, and in the inner ear. You can actually improve your hearing by pressing, rubbing, and massaging the indentation in the ear that faces your cheek. I have learned this from personal experience. When I was discharged from service in the military, I had deafness in my left ear which stayed with me for many years because of the compression of explosions I had witnessed in combat. Through this method of treatment and massage, I have regained most of my hearing and I now hear very well.

Next, I massage the upper part of my eyebrows cautiously (no heavy pressure). I use my middle and index fingers to work on the upper part of my eyelids with my eyes closed and massage the entire eyeball, and even below the eyeballs. Then I switch over and go into the middle part of my nostrils. On the outer part of my nose, I press right below the nasal bone that separates my eyes and give that a moderate massage. I then move down into the lower part of my eye where the big jawbones are and massage in there. I have a problem with sinus congestion, and this massage helps my sinuses immensely. These techniques are not necessarily a cure-all, but they do give you relief.

Using the fingertips of both hands, I massage my entire face, upper lip, lower lip, chin area, and around the lower part of the face skeleton. Continue the massage down to the Adam's apple and right below the indentations of your thyroid. If you massage this area with your fingertips, you will sometimes feel a little bit of a tickling sensation which has a beneficial effect on the thyroid.

At this point, I take two fingers and push up slightly on the end of my nose. I open up my eyes real wide and push my chin forward. It stretches a little bit of the nose and maintains the formation of the nostrils. For all of us in a degenerative state, everything on our bodies seems to be pulling down due to gravity. We need to keep pushing up, if you will. All of the movements that you make in your facial area should be a type of "pushing up." I do this little exercise with my nose twenty-five times in the morning. You push up gently, because if your nose looks good, your nostrils are pretty visible and you have a better-looking face. I have proven this through my own exercise program.

The next step is something you must do if you want to keep all the elasticity in your skin looking good. Without a doubt, the circulatory aspect of this massage is what causes the blood to flow into the skin area, making it look presentable and more youthful. I place four fingers on each side of my face. I start down at the lower part of my chin and push up very gently, all the way up to the top of my forehead. This is done ten times, pulling the skin and everything up very gently. Then I slowly push up the corners of my eyes toward my temples or toward the middle of my skull. I do that eight or ten times every morning. For the eye, I gently pull the very end on each side of the pupil over to the middle of my ear about ten times. I do these facial exercises every single morning before I get out of bed.

Next I massage the rest of my body. It takes about fifteen minutes in the morning, and if you take the time to try it, you'll see results. I guarantee it. In a thirty-day period, you'll have more beautiful skin texture and look a lot better. These are self-surgical procedures that are not done with any kind of doctors or surgeons. They help your appearance. You don't have to go through all the agony and pain of having a surgical facelift.

I also massage my feet every morning when I get up. Our feet take a huge beating each and every day because we walk on them. Gravity pulls our entire body down on our feet. During my morning routine, I briefly massage the end of each toe for four to ten seconds, and then I work all the way across each foot. You can press rather forcefully and massage a little at the indentations of your big toe on the bottom of your foot. This can help people with heart problems because it relates to the flow of blood around the muscle of the heart and improves circulation throughout your entire body.

Next you should move down into the inner side of each foot. After massaging the inner sides, use your thumbs to massage the middle of your foot, which is known as the inner part of your control system. After that, massage the entire heel and then move into the Achilles area of each foot. If you massage those parts of your feet, you'll experience a lot less arthritic pain and muscular aches. You can feel the benefits even if you're not having any problems at all. The massage can be performed just to keep the circulation going.

Along with the massage, I strongly recommend taking 120 milligrams (mgs) of the herb called *Ginkgo biloba* every morning. Ginkgo positively affects the circulatory system, including the heart and eyes. It can help prevent macular degeneration and heal tinnitus.

All of these preventative efforts take time and effort. If you don't take the time to practice them, you will not see the results. I've only learned this through experience. Most people think I look no more than fifty to fifty-five years of age, and that's quite a compliment. The only reason I'm this healthy is because I have taken these extra precautionary measures and have experienced their effectiveness.

When I have completed the foot massage, I lie down on the floor and stretch. I stretch every part of my body, reaching to the ceiling and taking deep breaths every time I move. I pull myself up with my arms and reach high above my head, stretching my entire body. I do this in a motion that is a little like kung fu in slow motion. I take that stretching exercise to the ceiling and drop it down to my chest area, where my hands are extended out in front of me. Then I do twenty-five knee bends. I inhale going down and exhale coming up.

Next I turn over on my stomach. I pull my arms as far out as they will go and stretch them up and stretch my legs out. I then pull up into a kneeling position with my arms and elbows on the floor. At this time, I cross my feet in such a way that my knees bend across my feet on each side, thus stretching them. After this, I straighten myself up in a camel-like arrangement with my butt in the air, and I pull with both legs to stretch my hip area at the waistline. If this is uncomfortable, you should stretch in a way that is more convenient for you.

You should keep your lungs in good shape because it is said that you are born with breath and you die without it. I suggest running up and down a stairwell two to four times each morning. This will help your breathing. When you are first starting, it will be an effort and you will find that your breathing is sometimes pretty intense and your heart is pumping hard, which is good.

Next, I always go out and run two to four miles. I've been doing this some fifty odd years and sometimes you get to a point where you are just completely exhausted. If this happens, I suggest that you take a couple of days off.

When you're doing aerobic exercises, sometimes you need a rest. Even my body occasionally gets to a point where I just can't do any more. I lay off for a while—a couple of days at the most.

There is another effective breathing exercise I would like to share with you. It involves standing up in a straight position, then reaching down with your legs straight, touching the floor, and grabbing hold of your toes on each foot. While grabbing your toes, take a deep breath and then bend your knees. Go down and then come back up, letting the air out. If you do this five times a couple of times a day, you will increase your breathing enormously.

There is another breathing exercise that involves holding your arms out to your sides as far as they will go. Make sure your arms are parallel to the floor. When you're doing this, bend over and stretch your arms back toward you, taking a deep breath. Then, take your arms and fold them back together with the palms of your hands. This will improve your breathing if you do it three or four times a day. You'll notice almost instantly how it helps.

Sometimes it's useful to have a little weight in each hand to hold out in front of you. Take a deep breath while you pull those weights out in an open position and come back in with the weights. While you are doing this, inhale while you are pulling the weights outward and exhale while the weights are coming back. This exercise also builds up your stomach muscles and helps if you have a weight problem.

Now I'd like to give you a little formula that I mix together *face cream*

and put on my face two or three times a day or in the evening that helps with the texture and glow of my skin. This formula makes a minimal amount, but can last two or three days if it's kept in the icebox. Start off by putting the white of an egg in a bowl, and pour about three or four tablespoons of organic soy milk on top of it. Then dissolve 3,000 mgs of vitamin C ascorbic acid in about a tablespoon full of water (this will take a few minutes). Once it's dissolved, throw it into the mixture. I also add a tablespoon of extra virgin olive oil. Then I take vitamin E capsules (400 international units, or IU) and penetrate the skin of the pills with a little needle or pricking point and squeeze them into the formula. I mix all of these components together in a small glass container and place a lid on it. Shake it up really well. The formula can be applied during the day if you don't have anything else to do, or can be applied in the evening before you go to bed. When you wake up in the morning, wash it off. The components of this formula are not really greasy because the egg helps to give texture to the skin and dries to a point where there is no stiffness.

This formula is very simple and inexpensive. It's a great alternative to going out and spending $150 to $250 for facial applications on the market. I guarantee that you will look better and your skin will look twenty-five years younger. This goes for young people and older people alike. You want to take care of your skin, and this is one way to do it. The formula I gave you should be applied to clean skin—that way it reaches all of the porous areas of your body.

I would also like to mention that I've always been a sun worshipper and I love to look tan. In my younger years, I probably tanned a little too much. Since I have an olive complexion, I don't burn too bad if I have enough sense to get out of the sun in time. If you have a lighter complexion, you need the sunshine because it provides a good amount of vitamin D. You definitely should try to expose yourself to the sun for short periods of time, so go out and enjoy the sunshine. It's good for you, but you also have to understand that you can burn, so be cautious! Vitamin E is an excellent sunscreen that also helps with burns.

I've noticed over time that many people have what is termed a "turkey neck." They have an excess amount of skin that is noticeable from the chin all the way down to the thyroid area. It's not a very attractive condition. However, it can be prevented with the facial exercises I gave you. Also, you can try to prevent or eliminate it by making a fist and placing it against the forehead. Put some pressure on your forehead and hold it for five seconds. Do this eight to ten times throughout the day. You can even do it when you're parked in a parking spot or waiting for a light to change. All of these methods are very effective in helping you improve the muscle tone in your face and entire body.

WEIGHT LOSS

Many claims exist about how people can lose weight. There are little simplistic approaches that not only help you lose weight, but which give your body both posture and definition. This healthy look is what we all should strive for. I'd like to talk to you about the necessity for and importance of exercising. Most people have a tendency to be sedentary. If you're not exercising, you're never going to achieve the type of body and mind and spirit that you're looking for. Exercise is the most essential thing that you can do.

While working at the pharmacy, I observed that most people, with the exception of very few, came in taking medications that were prescribed by their doctors practicing traditional medicine. I quizzed almost every single one of these people and learned that none of them exercised! They would often say, "It's too much effort, so I take a pill." That seems to be the traditional way in which people live. If my statistics are right (I believe that today it's even higher), only about 13% of the population actually exercises. That's a shame because you'll never be the person you want to be in mind, body, and spirit unless you exercise.

It doesn't have to be the exhausting type (I have experienced that through running marathons). As age creeps in and time goes by, marathons become even more difficult. You don't have the speed or endurance, but you're still in good shape and can do them. I have run fourteen marathons. I don't run them anymore, but I do run every day and sometimes even enjoy my run. There are times that I don't, but it takes effort every day. It should become a habit, for what you do habitually each and every day you continue to do. Then, if you don't, you feel guilty. Even if I'm tired, I go out and run and push myself. I exercise because it's become a habit, like brushing your teeth and cleaning your face in the morning. Exercise is the main ingredient in the success of your health.

Start immediately! Your exercise regimen does not have to be intense, and what you do when you first start out is something you should discuss with your practitioner. However, most doctors, I have found, make no suggestions at all. They do not ask if you exercise. The ones I've been to don't. They're too busy trying to get to the next patient and to make another buck, as far as I'm concerned. Many years ago I had a lot of faith in doctors, but I have very little in them now. If you've got a serious disease, yes, you need a diagnosis. You need to take your treatment into your own hands and decide how to deal with it. I have a son who had colon and prostate cancer and he elected not to go into the torture chamber (in my opinion) of chemotherapy. He's doing extremely well without it by taking alternative medicines. I'm not saying this will work for everybody, but if you do not want to go through the pain and agony of traditional medicines, it's certainly worth a try.

The big hype today, as everyone knows, is that people who are obese or overweight are taking an incredible amount of drugs. They are consuming substitutions and supplements of every nature and none of them seem to work as well as one would expect. People go to some drastic measures to lose weight, and yet there are some simplistic methods they can try. One of them is to take two teaspoons full of apple cider vinegar with each meal. Research has shown that a person can definitely lose weight by doing this, and it's good for just about any particular person. The size that you are or what you are eating doesn't make any difference. It seems as though the digestive track accepts the apple cider vinegar, helping to prevent extra weight and reducing the fatty cholesterol content in your body. You may ask your doctor about it, but in my opinion, it's better than taking Tagamet or the other antacids that are out there for your stomach. It works over a period of time, so don't expect to see the results immediately. It takes about two to three weeks to take effect, and like everything else that is being suggested here, it's not a miracle worker. These alternative medicines take time, working better over the length of time that you take them. Scientists have suggested that people who eat less live longer and are healthier. So remember when you take the vinegar that it counteracts your appetite and may even extend your life.

I believe that everyone, both men and women alike, is concerned about heart attacks. I have learned a great deal through my research, from my practitioners, and from all of the people in the vitamin and supplement business about how to prevent heart attacks. There are five essentials to explore and put into your body through your foods and supplementations. They are the A's, B's, C's, E's, and selenium. I want to put a little bit of emphasis on selenium. It is definitely, according to science and research, a real preventative. Research claims that people who take at least 200 micrograms (mcg) of selenium each and every day prevent their odds of having a heart attack by as much as 70%. It is something that you should really look into if you are not already taking it.

I am also a proponent of inflammatory supplements, especially as you grow older. There are many anti-inflammatory substances out there that do help. The medical profession insinuates that aspirin definitely helps people and protects a person from having another heart attack if they've already had one. Aspirin can serve as an anti-inflammatory which is very important for decreasing the risk of future heart attacks. One aspirin of 81 mgs a day doesn't have enough acidity to cause problems in most people. But taking a large amount of aspirin over a period of time, as you may well be aware, causes internal bleeding, and you must be careful if you are taking other forms of blood thinners. You certainly want to consult your doctor before taking aspirin.

DIETS

Now let's look at dieting. My weight-loss program is very effective. In fact, people can lose anywhere from three to eight pounds in three days by eating certain foods at certain times. I am going to relate to you some of the foods I recommend. For breakfast on day one, you should have black coffee or tea, one slice of toast, 1.5 cups of cereal (cold or hot), and half of a grapefruit. For lunch, eat one half-cup of tuna, a slice of toast, and coffee or tea. For dinner on day one, eat two slices (about three ounces) of any type of meat, one cup of broccoli, one cup of beets, one cup of low-fat frozen yogurt, and an apple. An apple a day keeps the doctor away, so they say.

On day two, breakfast consists of one egg, a slice of toast, black coffee or tea, and one apple. Lunch consists of one cup of cottage cheese, half of a banana, and five water crackers. You may not have heard of water crackers. They are not only palatable, but they're an item that is on the over-the-counter list in your favorite grocery store. For dinner on day two, you should have one skinless chicken breast, one cup of string beans, one half-cup of carrots, one half-cup of low-fat frozen yogurt, and a half of a banana. You should note that when I speak of yogurt, I'm talking about plain frozen yogurt, not the kind that has been infiltrated with all kinds of syrups and supposedly some kind of a fruit.

On day three, breakfast consists of a toasted bagel, one teaspoon of light cream cheese, 1.5 cups of cereal, one cup of black coffee or tea, and an apple. For lunch, eat one boiled egg, one slice of toast, and a small salad with one tablespoon of light dressing. Dinner on day three should consist of one cup of tuna, one cup of beets, one cup of fresh broccoli, and one half-cup of low-fat frozen yogurt. For dessert you can have half of a cantaloupe or something else in that category of fruit.

The suggestion for best results is to have a daily elimination in large quantities. Fresh fruits, dried fruits, prune juice or prunes, and psyllium husks (not the powder) will accelerate elimination. I strongly recommend the psyllium husks. You can buy them at the health food store and put them in your favorite juice to help cleanse your body and reduce cholesterol. After the husks have been consumed, you should drink a glass of water immediately. In fact, drink a glass of water at least six times a day. Water enhances elimination and flushes fat.

The dieter may not only experience a loss of weight, but will also be addressing other health issues. Doctors recommend getting your daily allowance of nutrients and more of the antioxidants that may prevent free radical damage that causes clogged arteries, heart disease, and lung disease, among others. This diet is proven to work on chemical breakdown. Do not vary or substitute any of the above foods. Pepper may be used in moderation, and where there aren't any dietary restrictions. Allowing for common-sense variations, the diet should be followed three days at a time. In three days, you can lose up to eight pounds. After three days of dieting, you may eat normal food, but do not overdo it. After four days of normal eating, you can start back on your three-day diet.

As with any diet, please contact your physician and get his advice about exercise and fluid intake. The diet suggestions of foods to reduce fat intake are: ice milk, low-fat yogurt, slim or skim milk, water crackers, pumpkin seeds with no salt, fish, omega-3 fatty acids, a dry bagel, light meals, and angel food cake. Those on the non-acceptable list are: ice cream, sour cream, whole milk, salt crackers, salted nuts, fatty meats, croissants, dark meats, and pound cake. All of these foods contain an enormous amount of fat.

Individual weight may vary. There are some people who lose up to eight pounds in three days by following the above diet, but as with any weight-loss program, sensible eating habits will contribute to your success. I've done an enormous amount of research over a period of three years about this particular diet. Give it a shot because I know it will work. Satisfaction is guaranteed if you follow the instructions, and it works in the way that nature intended. It is not to be done in the harsh ways that some people are putting themselves through in order to lose weight.

Here are few items that are store-bought or are from fast food restaurants that you must avoid if you intend to reduce your weight problem and acquire more energy. Tucker Ridge Farms Original Flaky Chicken Pot Pie, believe it or not, has 500 calories and 9 grams of saturated fat. When you look at the label again, you realize that the numbers are for just half of the pie. If you eat the whole pie, as most people probably do, you are consuming more than 1000 calories and 18 grams of saturated fat. When you add the 13 grams of hidden trans fat from the partially hydrogenated vegetable shortening in each pie, you are up to 31 grams of artery-clogging fat. That's more than a day's allotment and isn't good for your heart.

Another bad choice would be McDonald's Select Premium Chicken Breast Strips. They sound healthy, but in fact, the chicken strips are no healthier than the chain's Chicken McNuggets. A standard five-strip order has 630 calories and 11 grams of artery-clogging fat. That's about the same as a Big Mac, except the burger has 110 mgs of sodium. Another factory reject would be a slice of the Cheesecake Factory's 6 Carb Original Cheesecake. It has 610 calories, which is the same amount of calories in a slice of the Original Cheesecake. Think of it as eating an eight ounce prime rib steak for dessert that has 29 grams of saturated fat—a one-and-a-half-day's supply. The next time you step on the bathroom scale, you may never know that the carbohydrates were missing.

Dove Ice Cream squeezes 300 calories and anywhere from 9-13 grams of saturated fat (that's half a day's worth) into a half-cup serving of ice cream. That puts it in the same ballpark as Ben & Jerry's and Häagen-Dazs. With names like Unconditional Chocolate, Dove is trying to entice you with romance. A scoop of its ice cream will fill your heart all right, but not with love. Who would guess that a single Mrs. Fields Milk Chocolate and Walnut Cookie would have more than 300 calories and as much saturated fat as a twelve ounce sirloin steak? It also has six teaspoons of sugar.

Let's now take a look at coffee. Starbucks' Strawberries and Cream Frappuccino with whipped cream is more than a mere cup of sugar. Think of it as a milkshake. Few people have room in their diets for 770 calories and 19 grams of fat, ten of which are saturated. That is half a day's quota. Every cup supplies this amount. It's like the nutritional equivalent of a Pizza Hut Personal Pan Pepperoni Pizza that you sip through a straw. Watch out!

Burger King should be called the Coronary King. They serve some of the most harmful French fries you can buy. A king-sized order packs 600 calories and 75% of your daily maximum diet for your heart. They are very unhealthy.

One of the things that concerns me about Campbell's soups is that you can rarely find one of their products that does not contain MSG. MSG, as you know, is a preservative and is extremely hard on your system. It reminds me a lot of Chinese food. In many instances, Chinese restaurants serve an enormous amount of MSG. It tastes good so that's why they have it in their products. Moreover, Campbell's red-and-white-label condensed soups are brimming with salt. Half a can averages more than half a person's daily quota of salt. Instead, try brands like Healthy Choice and Campbell's Healthy Requests, which have less than half as much sodium.

Swoops are the essence of your favorite chocolate candy, thus explains the packaging. The unique shape envelopes your mouth in chocolate. Hershey's bars contain almost 200 calories and 7-8 grams of saturated fat. That's one-third of a day's worth, as well as more than four teaspoons of sugar. A Mint Chip Dazzler at Häagen-Dazs includes three scoops of ice cream, hot fudge, Oreos, chocolate sprinkles, and whipped cream. That's 1,270 calories and 38 grams of saturated fat, which is two days' worth of your saturated fats! Think of it as a portable T-bone steak with a Caesar salad and a baked potato with sour cream. That's a dinner, yet many people have a dazzler as dessert after they've eaten both lunch and dinner.

Those snacks contain an enormous amount of saturated fat. You should stay away from them completely. Read the labels on the foods you want at the store. Any processed foods are going to be unhealthy. Be very cautious if you're interested in maintaining a healthy diet.

On the other side of the spectrum, one of the super foods for better health is sweet potatoes. One example is a nutritional All-

Star, which is one of the best sweet potatoes you can eat. It's loaded with carotenoids, vitamin C, and fiber. Mix unsweetened applesauce or crushed pineapple with the sweet potato to give it extra moisture and sweetness. White potatoes have a lot of potassium, but they do raise your insulin level by 30%. After you eat a white potato, you might become hyper. Tomatoes are a good source of flavonoids, which are excellent for your prostate and help prevent cancer. Tomatoes' little bite-size shape makes them perfect for dipping or eating in salads. They are packed with phytochemicals, vitamins C and E, and some fiber.

Fat-free or 1% milk, but not 2%, is an excellent source of calcium, vitamins, and protein. There are no artery-clogging fats or cholesterol. Soy milk can be just as nutritious if it's added to something you eat. If you spill any of it on your hands, just rub it all over your face. Soy milk is excellent for your complexion. Blueberries are rich in fiber, vitamin C, and antioxidants. Eat them in cereal or stir them in yogurt. Don't buy yogurt with blueberries because it contains a lot of added sugar. You can also sprinkle blueberries over low-fat ice cream.

Whole-grain rye crackers like Wasa, Rye Krisp, and Rye Vieda, usually called crisp breads, are fat-free and loaded with fiber. Eat brown rice only. Enriched white rice is bankrupt of all nutrition. You lose the fiber, magnesium, vitamins E and B6, copper, and zinc that you get in brown rice. Who knows what phytochemicals are in the whole-grain rice that you miss when buying white rice, so try the brown rice instead.

Citrus fruits taste great, and they're rich in vitamin C, folic acid, and fiber. They're perfect for a snack and dessert. Try dessert varieties, such as juicy Mineola oranges, clementines, or a tart grapefruit. Every morning, I squeeze half a lemon into a glass with two ounces of Aloe vera gel. I then top it off with about six to eight ounces of grape juice. This makes an excellent nutritional drink. It helps with constipation and gives you energy. If you are a runner like I am, you could drink it every morning before you run and have more energy.

What about squash? Grocery stores provide squash that is peeled, seeded, sliced, as well as microwaveable. I personally do not like to use the microwave only because of the radiation. I don't need that and you don't, either. If you buy these products in a container, be cautious because of the spinach scare not too long ago. It is always best to buy whole squash. Any time something is cut up, it always has the possibility of containing some bacteria. Thoroughly wash everything that comes in a precut bag, including greens.

Greens like kale, spinach, and broccoli are nutritional powerhouses. Most are loaded with vitamin C, carotenoids, calcium, folic acid, potassium, and fiber. Now it's easy to squeeze the greens into your busy schedule. You should be aware of the good and the bad of what you purchase when you go to the grocery store.

FOOD INTAKE

All of the concepts in this book revolve around anti-aging. Being eighty years old, I have lived a long life and experienced a tremendous amount of tension, a negative feeling you want to avoid. I started my education through medical (traditional) doctors, only to discover that nothing I took at their suggestion did anything but put me on the floor. It just knocked me out and completely annihilated my thought processes. It did not matter if I took small or large doses. One of the things I could never understand about doctors was that when they prescribed something (I am not a big man at 5'9" and 145 pounds), they gave me the same dosage as a person who weighed 300 pounds. It never did make sense to me, but that is their thinking.

Let's go on with thoughts of anti-aging, living longer, feeling better, and preventing the diseases that are trying to haunt us each and every day. First of all, I have mentioned before that one of the greatest things you should be doing for your body is putting fiber in it. I have found that the best time to consume fiber is in the morning. The greatest sources are plant foods that are good for you and high in fiber content. New findings indicate that eating fiber early in the day is particularly helpful because it prevents spikes of blood sugar and glucose that can damage arteries and increase the risk of fatty buildup and heart disease. You should eat fiber at breakfast to slow the rate at which the stomach empties. It increases bowel movements so that you are less likely to snack and gain excessive calories later.

Fiber-rich foods include something as easy as Kellogg's All-Bran Cereal. It has 10 grams of fiber per half cup. Raspberries and other fruits count as well. Every kind of berry is excellent for good fiber. New findings point out that people who drink large amounts of green tea, which is rich in flavonoids, have lower rates of breast and prostrate cancer. I have tried green tea many times. As I've mentioned, I cannot handle too much caffeine, and green tea has caffeine. Some caffeine is good for you, but I can't handle much because of my increased heart rate. Thus, I have tried to stay away from it, although I drink it periodically. If you can handle caffeine, green tea is one of the best things you can possibly do for your body. It will give you the necessary ingredients for a healthy heart. Green tea contains vitamins C and E and other bioflavonoids. It is suggested that you take 31 mgs in three to four cups a day. Even with the consumption of these ingredients, it is still suggested that you take supplements. As I mentioned before, I take 4,000 to 5,000 mgs of vitamin C alone and 400 to 800 mgs of vitamin E every single day.

EYES

What can go wrong with our eyes? Diseases that afflict the eyes include cataracts, glaucoma, macular degeneration, myopia, and hyperopia. Many treatments and preventions have been developed over the years for these eye illnesses. Vitamin A can help relieve eye discomfort, or in some cases, even heal your eyes.

Cataracts

A cataract develops when the lens of the eye becomes fogged due to either a decrease in fluids surrounding the lens, poor circulation, or nutritional deficiency. Cataracts impair the detail of a person's vision by causing a haze and preventing light from penetrating the lens. This condition tends to get worse over time, even to the point of blindness in the most extreme cases. Cataracts affect either one or both eyes.

Glaucoma

Glaucoma, similar to cataracts, is caused by glandular loss of sight initially affecting a person's peripheral vision. The optic nerve is quite sensitive and can be damaged by fluid, sunlight, infection, circulatory problems, and exposure to toxins. Glaucoma pressure in the eye tends to progressively increase, damaging the optic nerve. This causes gradual vision loss, and without proper care, can develop into blindness.

Macular Degeneration

Macular degeneration is another primary cause of blindness. It is a condition that occurs when a tiny area of the central retina called the macula deteriorates. Macular degeneration happens primarily in the elderly. It occurs for a variety of reasons, such as nutritional deficiencies, circulatory problems, and arterial sclerosis. Exposure to electrical magnetic fields through heavy computer use can also contribute to this condition.

Myopia

This condition is generally referred to as nearsightedness. The eye brings light into focus before it hits the retina, which results in difficulty seeing objects that are far away.

Hyperopia

Hyperopia is the opposite of myopia. Light is brought into focus behind the retina, thus causing objects at a close range to appear blurry. In the case of glaucoma, there are additional symptoms that include headache, eye pain, redness in the eyes, nausea, vomiting, and abnormally wide pupils.

Eye Treatments

Some of the conventional treatments for these illnesses, such as surgery, don't generally have a whole lot of success. There are many side effects from surgery. Muscles in and around the eyes tend to worsen, and some people still need to rely on prescriptive lenses to improve vision. Nutrition has had an enormously high rate of success in regards to eye problems. The nutrients associated with proper eye care are vitamins E and D. The general maintenance of healthy eyes is associated with vitamin A for proper liver metabolism and digestion, and vitamin C for ridding the bloodstream of toxins. Also of value are glutathione for helping rid the eye of excess fluid, selenium, carotenoids, and niacin for increasing circulation. All of the B vitamins, the omega-3 fatty acids found in fish oil for decreasing inflammation, and a balance of magnesium and calcium for proper muscle control are helpful.

All of these nutrients can be taken in the form of supplements. These ingredients can also be found in a vegetarian diet and are a great way to get the proper nutrients for eye care. Carrots, green leafy vegetables (such as beet greens, spinach, and broccoli), and yellow, green, and orange fruits (particularly in the form of fresh organic fruit juice) are a great source of vitamin A. Furthermore, sulfur-rich foods, such as eggs, garlic, and asparagus, increase the amount of C and E in the body. There are some herbs like Ginkgo biloba and hawthorne berry that help immensely. They increase circulation and create the same effect as common spices, such as marjoram, cayenne pepper, ginger, and garlic.

Bilberry is an excellent nutrient for night vision. When I was in the military, we would take a couple of tablespoons of bilberry jelly before we took off at nighttime. It was amazing how our nighttime focusing improved. Grape seed extract can be used to fortify the capillaries that furnish the eye with fluids and aid in the prevention of lens impairment. Recommended dosages are 120 to160 mgs a day.

There are certain exercises that can be beneficial in correcting particular conditions. Daily activity is recommended to help lower intraocular pressure and increase circulation. This can be done with a brisk walk or exercising in general. A more enhancing exercise for peripheral vision is to imagine a clock. In visualizing the clock, rotate the eyes counterclockwise from twelve to nine and back again. Then move the eyes in the opposite direction from twelve to three and back. This should be done without the help of corrective eyewear and using a thumb as a guide during the exercise. The person should be attentive to the objects along the perimeter of the scope of vision. This drill can be done three times a day or more to strengthen the muscles in and around the eyes. Also, stop and take deep breaths until the sight becomes clearer and the object can be brought in closer again, and then repeat.

Another muscle-strengthening exercise involves sitting in the middle of the room. Gaze up to the ceiling and then down following the visual path of a straight line to the floor. This can be repeated several times. The same process should be done looking from one side of the room to the other. Deep breathing should be performed during the exercise to release tension in the eyes. While in a comfortable position, cover the eyes with the palm of the hands and visualize a peaceful place that gives you serenity while breathing deeply. Also, massage can increase circulation to the neck and subsequently to the eyes.

Another great therapeutic procedure is acupuncture. A qualified practitioner of acupuncture can do wonders for all parts of the body, including the eyes. Needles are used to stimulate particular parts of the eye and thus improve your vision. A couple of visits to a good practitioner can be beneficial for people who are having eye problems. It is definitely something to be considered.

What should you avoid? Particular foods and environmental factors can be harmful to the eyes, resulting in vision impairment. These include artificial sweeteners, for they contain toxic substances that can negatively affect the optic nerve. Caffeine affects circulation, alcohol can damage liver function, and sugar may hinder enzyme function. Also, you should avoid lactose (a form of sugar found in dairy products), tobacco, steroids, and the toxins and mercury found in dental amalgam. Fillings and exposure to direct sunlight can cause oxidative damage to the eyes.

In brief, treatment should include vitamins A, C, D, and E, gluthianone, selenium, carotenoids, niacin, and all of the B vitamins. Also to be included are omega-3 fatty acids, Ginkgo biloba, hawthorne berry, and the proper balance of magnesium and calcium. The field of vision therapy offers exercises and lifestyle advances that can help strengthen the eyes. Daily activity is important to help lower intraocular pressure and increase circulation. Acupuncture, reflexology, bio-feedback, and other techniques can improve vision. Hopefully all of the above can benefit you in your lifetime of sight.

Footnote to vitamin A: Beta-carotene is a precursor of vitamin A and thus can be taken in larger quantities without any negative side effects. One of the side effects of taking excessive vitamin A is jaundice, which is the yellowing of the skin and eyes. Therefore, precautionary measures should be followed when taking vitamin A. It is excellent for you as long as it's not taken in great quantities. Up to 50,000 IU of beta-carotene can be taken per day without any adverse effects.

SKIN

I want to talk about another important subject matter: skin. Soothing sensitive skin is essential for good health. Allergists, dermatologists, and other people who treat your skin have made many suggestions about skin health. For the number of times I have been to dermatologists, most of them have been in awe of some of my suggestions about relieving dry skin problems. Sometimes allergies cause you to sneeze and make you itch. But don't worry, you can find relief. The itchiness might begin a short time after something is placed on the skin.

For instance, if you have a new ring on your finger and you're unaware of the fact that you may be allergic to the metal, irritation could begin around the ring. In this situation, you might not know what's causing your problem. I have allergies and I have never had a reaction to a metal as far as I can recall, but some of the problems that people experience are with metals. If metals bother you, you can treat your skin in several different ways. Topical skin applications might help, and you may want to try them before you attempt to see a dermatologist or an allergist. Contaminating contact skin allergies, known formally as allergic contact dermatitis, vary in severity depending on what type of sensitivity you have. Redness may clear up with soap and water, or may progress into skin-damaging sores. You want to wash them and keep them clean or you could continue to have bad reactions if you have sensitivity to metals.

You have to work with your dermatologist to determine what is causing your skin problem. Sometimes seemingly harmless sea water, cement, shoe leather, soil, or blue pottery can cause unsightly and painful rashes. Allergies to metal and other topical irritants are so common that more than 54% of the population had a positive skin test response to one or more allergies, according to the *Journal of Clinical Immunology.* Often allergies can develop out of seemingly nowhere. I have seen it happen with my clients. One day, without warning, they develop a metal allergy. Sometimes an eye shadow or a fabric softener can cause an outbreak. If the inflammatory substance histamine is released, hives may appear and become extremely itchy. While more common among adults, allergic dermatitis is the most widespread of skin conditions.

In children younger than eleven, the percentage of kids diagnosed with skin ailments continues to increase. Why the jump in allergic skin reactions? The problem is that an ever-increasing number of chemical substances come into contact with our bodies. The increasing popularity of body piercings has resulted in metal allergies in places you never dreamed of. A surge of trendy yet chemically laden beauty products, topical drugs, and sometimes even detergents, soaps, and lotions add to the fuel of the itchy fire. I find that people who have allergic reactions also tend to catch colds and the flu more easily, are likely to have a history of asthma or eczema, and tend to get fatigued more easily. Moderate amounts of exercise and maybe an acupuncturist or herbalist can help. In traditional Chinese medicine, which views the body more as a collection of functions than a collection of organs, the skin is considered to be associated with the lungs. Both the skin and lungs serve as a line of defense against outside influences.

Many people who have skin allergies will also suffer from upper respiratory illness. The body's defense against diseases of this nature is a Chinese word called Gi. Gi results in allergic reactions when a person has been exposed to something like dampness that causes an imbalance and disturbs the flow of energy throughout the body. This results in itching, red blotches, or seeping lesions. When treating someone for allergies, the practitioner must pay attention to the constitution of the patient and to how the allergic symptoms present themselves. Herbs are given in Chinese medicine to nourish the Gi.

One of the arsenals of defense is a product the Chinese often prescribe called Astragalus. It is an immune regulator and is also used to prevent upper respiratory infections. Sometimes Astragalus is recommended for people who have an allergic reaction and don't know the cause. There are simple things that you should change, like your approach to washing, detergents, and such. Discontinue the use of products that are suspected to be causing the reaction. If you need to scratch, it is okay to scratch around the area. Just be careful that your fingernails do not touch the infected area because they have a poisonous effect on it.

Sometimes folk remedies are beneficial to inflamed skin. A topical application of apple cider vinegar with a paste of sea salt and water can help the skin, and if the skin is dry, use a hypoallergenic moisturizer. Test everything on a small area first to see if it's acceptable to your skin. There are herbs that can cool fiery-feeling skin. An herbalist trained in healthcare can recommend many different proven remedies. One of those suggestions might include an anti-inflammatory product called burdock. Another herb called calendula boosts the immune system. All of these can be bought at your health food store.

There are natural antiseptics that can be applied topically as a lotion ointment, like cooling aloe gel or lotion. I'm familiar with Aloe vera gel because I use it on my face. Remember, I have been told over and over again how beautiful my skin is for my age! I not only put it on topically, but I take a couple of ounces internally, especially when my stomach is upset. I still think that most of our problems are based on what we put into our stomachs, and food allergies have a major impact on our health and our skin.

There are various anti-inflammatory treatments that are being suggested. You can make a paste out of a product called goldenseal root or peppermint oil, which soothes a burn. Soothing problems on the outside can be added to what you take internally. Be sure you get all the nutrients you need, especially the omega-3 fatty acids, B vitamin complex, and vitamin C. You can also try eliminating a lot of your wheat products. Some people are not aware that many products we buy at the store are contaminated with wheat and wheat gluten. When I substituted wheat with rice and rice-made products over a period of a few months, I saw a drastic improvement in my overall wellbeing and especially in my skin. For some individuals, skin allergies are a huge part of their lives, be it identifying allergies, relieving symptoms, or avoiding allergens. For others, an occasional outbreak is nothing more than an itchy nuisance. Try filling your medicine chest and utility closet with non-allergenic, fragrance-free items, including makeup and beauty products. You should choose proper dish detergents and house cleaners as well.

When you are having these problems with your skin, it's important to keep your bowels open. This can be done in several ways, such as by drinking prune juice and eating prunes. You can try dates and many of the products out there that give you natural elimination. For those of you that have a lot of problems with your skin, be sure to always use sunscreen.

One of the most maddening forms of allergies is hives. These large, itchy bumps can be treated in many ways that we have mentioned above. Again, it is very important to take a multivitamin and a high-potency multivitamin. Try to acquire 3,000 mgs of vitamin C and 200 to 400 IU of vitamin E. There are other fighters out there, too, which are used to digest enzymes. One of them is bromelain, taken three times a day with meals. When an outbreak occurs, you should be taking 100 mgs of each B vitamin four times a day, along with two herbs of bilberry, 60 mgs, three times a day. Another product that I strongly encourage you to take every single day is called stinging nettles. Take one capsule every two to four hours. Mix with a liquid beta-carotene, which is a precursor to vitamin A.

FACE

I want to elaborate on things that you can do specifically for your face. There's one thing I keep in my bathroom and apply to my face in the morning and evening. I take 3,000 mgs of vitamin C ascorbic acid and put it in two to three ounces of water. I let it dissolve and shake it up, and then apply it to my face. It's excellent for people who have chronic acne and also helps maintain the elasticity in your skin.

MASSAGE

Forehead and eyes: Take four fingers on both hands and place them on your forehead. Pressing gently, move the skin in an up, down, and around movement. These moves stimulate blood flow. Then take the index finger of both hands and apply to the top of your eyelids. Very gently press, with your eyes closed, over the upper and lower eyes for a few seconds. Next, apply the palms of your hands over your closed eyes for about ten seconds. This definitely improves eyesight.

Ears: As everyone is aware, the ears are those odd-looking wing-like objects on the sides of the head. They hopefully let us hear what's going on around us. Did you know that different areas of the ear have some connection with all of our body parts? Massaging our ears helps healing. For example, by pinching your ear lobes, you relieve tension and stress as well as improve eyesight. Therefore, massaging your ears in the morning is quite beneficial to your health. It's one of my favorite activities to do while driving.

Nose: Rubbing the framework of your nose can prevent a number of maladies. Living in an area like mine, sinus problems with allergies are extremely common. You simply place your fingers on the bridge of the nose and apply slight pressure while massaging. This will help the sinuses drain. Also, every morning I irrigate my sinuses with saline solution. It's nothing but a mixture of one-fourth teaspoon baking soda and one-half teaspoon sea salt in four ounces of pure boiled water. Holding my head between my knees and squirting the solution with an atomizer three or four times fills the nose canal. Once this is done, hold your head down for one or two minutes. This allows the saline solution to enter the sinus area. If you sniff it into the sinus area, that will help it to penetrate further. I've found through personal experience that this procedure almost always prevents sinus infections. As I know from working in a pharmacy for years, this practice was suggested to many patients who suffered continuous sinus infections.

Another approach for sinus relief is an herb that's not too well-known. It is called stinging nettles. I have tried most suggested relief potions, both over-the-counter and prescription. Nettles give relief without the side effects that most of the more popular solutions seem to cause.

Many people have asked, "What do you do to keep looking so young?" My response is that it's just habit! People might think that it's hard work. Not true. The following is a routine I've practiced daily for years. After waking at about 7:00 a.m., being a God-fearing man, I pray for good health and the care of my six children and their mother. I then proceed to massage my face with my fingers in bed, gently rubbing for about five minutes. I massage my forehead, eyes, ears, nose, cheeks, jaw bones, lips, chin, and all around my neck. This stimulates the blood flow. I put a finger on my nose and push up gently. I then open my eyes and mouth while pushing my nose up to keep my skin firm. Before exiting my bed, I sit on its edge and put my feet up one at a time on my knee, massaging the bottom and top of both feet. This is called reflexology. It stimulates your entire body. Each section of the bottom of your feet has places that connect with certain parts of your body.

For circulation and healing, my next approach is to drink one full glass of water. With this water, I take two acidophilus tablets, which represents more than two billion strains of good flora. Also, I swallow 1,000 mgs of vitamin C, 400 IU of vitamin E, beta-carotene, B100, selenium, and many others. These are very synergistic.

It is important to have good bowel elimination at least two times a day. This is facilitated by taking one heaping tablespoon of pure psyllium husk, purchased at health food stores. I mix powdered kelp, ginger, glucosamine, and chondroitin (liquid) with the psyllium. Then I add a heaping tablespoon of creatine formula, which includes taurine, glutamine, and L-arginine. This can be taken with good fruit juice—I use prune juice. Taken with a large glass of water, this mixture helps the psyllium husk to work the bowel more efficiently. In my opinion, this may be the key to all good health. Many health experts preach that you should have two to three eliminations per day.

My next move is to stretch for a good five minutes. Over the eighty years of my life, exercising has become a habit. Before I run every day, I stretch my whole body for at least five minutes. Then I proceed to run, regardless of the weather, three to four miles. After running fourteen marathons, which equal 26.2 miles,

I got worn out. Now I mostly do shorter runs. At this time in my life, marathons are too hard on my body.

After my run, my breakfast consists of at least two or three fruits, raw or cooked, placed on cereal. If you're looking for great health, remember to read the label on every product to determine its contents. A great number of cereals are loaded with sugar and whole wheat, so most of my cereals are composed of Quaker raw oats, which are great for good cholesterol. Since protein is so very essential, four or five eggs do a great job each week. I enjoy poached eggs on grain toast with honey. It creates a good tasting formula with caffeine-free green tea. I prefer caffeine-free because I don't want to risk having an irregular heartbeat. Chocolate and other products with caffeine do not agree with some people and I am one of them. I also consume a large glass of water. Drinking seven to eight glasses of distilled water per day ensures good health.

Don't forget that this God-given body we have is one great plumbing system. Water pushes the many toxins we accumulate out of our body each day. This kind of elimination is no secret. It just has to happen. If you're not ingesting seven to eight glasses of water a day, then begin to do so now. You will see a dramatic improvement in every part of your body, especially in your skin. I carry a gallon of water in my car to make sure I do not forget its importance.

Over the years everyone experiences different types of foods and exercises that their body can tolerate. This is where my vitamins and supplements have kept me healthy, vibrant, and young.

As I have mentioned earlier, I had to figure this out the hard way. You need to know that I have pushed my body and mind.

This man enjoys smoking a cigar a day, along with drinking a couple of alcoholic beverages. If these things doesn't agree with you or you disapprove of them, then you don't have to do them.

I consume about seventy supplements and vitamins a day. The intent of this book is to explain why I take them. The results of my research will prove, without a doubt, the effectiveness of what I take. The time of day is important to note when taking vitamins. Vitamin E supplements are very synergistic when taken together with doses of vitamin C and D-alpha-tocopheryl. I have found that a therapeutic dose of 3,000 to 4,000 mgs of vitamin C per day does wonders for my immune system. You should take vitamin C in 1,000 mg increments four or five times a day. Most of our ascorbic acid (vitamin C) is lost when we have a bowel elimination and urine release. Some is also lost as we perspire. Thus, taking vitamin C in intervals protects our immune system.

Many practitioners have written that vitamin C may prevent some cancers and heart problems. It suppresses cold and flu symptoms, aiding the immune system to fight off the virus. Many doctors tell their patients that vitamin C only gives them expensive urine. Please don't believe that! If you ever need information on the health benefits of vitamin C, read the confirmation from Linus Pauling. He was an acclaimed Nobel Prize winner twice. He professes the importance of vitamin C to health. How could any medical man contradict such a man as Dr. Pauling? He spent many of his ninety-three years proving the importance of vitamin C and its gift to society for better health.

BREATHING

It has been said that we are born with breath and we die without it. When your lungs become inflamed from flu, colds, or lack of energy, it might be associated with all the toxins and bad food you're putting into your stomach. This may cause breathing problems. Breathing problems are sometimes an indication that the heart is not functioning properly, or are a result of lack of exercise and good nutritional foods.

I worked at a pharmacy for eleven years and I have seen so many patients coming in for their medications for bronchitis and emphysema. Breathing problems can be caused by many different things. However, all the medications in the world won't replace exercise.

Of course, along with exercise, relaxing is an important factor. If you do nothing to control yourself, stress can damage your emotional and physical wellbeing. It can harm a relationship. When you find you're getting tired and stressed out, take a fifteen-minute break and meditate. I do this every single day because I get extremely tired sometimes. Take a break and close your eyes. Just sit or lie comfortably with your eyes closed. Slowly count backwards from ten to one. Work on obtaining the feeling that your toes and feet are relaxing, and then your legs, your diaphragm, your stomach, your heart and your lungs, your chest and throat, your chin and your eyes and nose, your sinuses and ears. They all need to be relaxed.

I am also a certified hypnotherapist. I help people to relax, stop smoking, lose weight, etc. I find that meditation is extremely helpful. I have seen so many people in my practice who have started doing breathing exercises come back to tell me that their breathing has improved 100%, and they feel much better and continue to do it.

There are certain supplements that help along the way. One of them is definitely vitamin E at 400 to 800 IU a day. This is a preferable amount when starting out your exercise program for your lungs. The omega-3 fatty acids, fish oils (that contain flax), and borage oils are a combination of nutrients you can get at your health food store. They should be taken in units of 3,000 mgs per day. With the fish oils, I prefer a combination of flax seed, borage oils, and fish oils. Most of these fish oils contain many ingredients such as RNA and DNA, which are the amino acids that help with breathing. Fish oil lubricates the lungs and helps with many other areas. One supplement that I personally take is stinging nettles. Take as directed and they will work wonders for your breathing and also help your immune system immensely.

Garlic is another great supplement. Garlic is good for just about everything, but it definitely helps in the lung area. All of these ingredients can be taken as suggested by their labels. If you are not getting results after taking a supplement for about thirty days, you may try increasing the dosage or substituting it with something else.

So to sustain a high quality of life and live longer, don't forget to learn how to breathe. Some people just take it for granted. And that's okay until it starts hindering you. If you have sinuses and allergies, you might have some form of breathing problems because mucus hinders breathing. Certain foods agitate your breathing, and then the agitation becomes inflammatory. These are things you have to figure out yourself. Not even doctors can tell you unless you have an allergy test taken. Sometimes doctors find the problem and sometimes they don't. So it is your problem and you have to find out what foods and other materials cause your allergies and breathing problems. It is a time-consuming process, but eventually you will diagnose your problems and you will feel much better. Good luck. I had a problem with this for many years and found some of the things that I just suggested helped me more than anything else. I suggest trying them and seeing what will work. If you want to feel better, then it is something you have to do.

DIGESTIVE TRACT

I am personally affected by this next issue. In my opinion and in the research that I have done over many years, I have found that people who do not have good eliminations (I am talking about two to three bowel eliminations every single day), have problems. People not only have problems with constipation, but can also develop diseases of many kinds if constipation is not taken care of.

Most of my life I was constipated. Even in the navy, I remember having a hard time with my bowels. I am a stressed-out man. When I say stressed out, I mean I just seem to have a hard time relaxing. Those people who are more relaxed and exercise and do the things they are supposed to do to help stimulate bowel elimination every day have better results because they are so relaxed. There are so many things out there that can help you, and there is one that I learned about and have suggested to many of my patients.

A product called psyllium husks, taken as a huge tablespoon each and every day with your favorite juice, is a great help. I personally take mine with prune juice. Psyllium is an expanding type of grain. You should drink a couple of glasses of water after you have taken it because it expands in your stomach. If you don't drink water, it seems to give you a lot of indigestion. I don't suggest that you do this every single morning, but if you have a problem with constipation, you can do this for a couple of weeks. Please note that I am talking about psyllium husks and not the powder. The powder has a bad effect on some people.

Psyllium has been a great success for the people I've suggested it to. They came in with high cholesterol, and after two months, it had gone down to normal. No more drugs. That made them happy and made me happy knowing that they followed my suggestion and it worked.

Some people never try taking psyllium and want to go along with the doctor who is just going to give them some form of medication that will enhance a bowel movement. But you can do this naturally. Along with taking psyllium and prune juice and water in the morning, I eat anywhere from four to six stewed prunes. You should do this before you eat breakfast. They don't have to be stewed; you can eat them raw. If you like them, they are an excellent product. Prunes have all forms of minerals, iron, and protein, and they contain many of the good carbohydrates. They are excellent for your physical wellbeing. They even enhance brain power and give you energy. You can eat them as a snack if you want. I wouldn't suggest eating them all day long because you will be visiting the bathroom too often. But this type of approach will give you a bowel movement two to three times a day.

In fact, most gastroenterologists agree that you should have two to three bowel movements per day in order to have a healthy digestive and bowel system. They claim it should have no odor to speak of. For a long time, I didn't agree with that, but I do agree now. I find that by doing what I just suggested, my stools do not smell or have that offensive odor. You may pass some gas throughout the day and that is good. I think the estimated number of times for most people to release gas during the day is somewhere around fifteen to twenty times or more. This is imperative for good health because everything that you put into your stomach must come out.

Sometimes I am in a restaurant and eat something that is not very good for me, especially pork. Pork, it has been said and written, is the worst food you can eat. You cannot cook or boil all of the bacteria out of this particular meat. Be cautious about pork, and be careful about eating fatty meats of any kind. It is suggested, if you have the opportunity, to eat nothing but wild game, such as deer, rabbit, squirrel, and wild fish. Always be sure that the fish you eat were wild in nature, and not farmed. It has been proven that most farmed fish are not healthy because they eat each other's fecal matter. So be cautious in that respect. As far as elimination is concerned, fruits, vegetables, and organic cereals help immensely. You should also consider buying organic foods. It is a little more expensive, but in the long run, your health is worth it. Make sure that most of the things you buy are in an organic state, especially your fruits and vegetables. They are offered in many places now. I've been seeing organic foods in the big chain stores because it is becoming such a popular thing. That will again help you with your eliminations.

One of the beautiful things about having these eliminations each and every day is how they affect your health. I am amazed that when people regulate their bowels, their health improves immensely. If you are on medications and drugs, you can rest assured that it will be tough to get back. You may, after a period of time following the instructions above, be able to eradicate or get rid of some of the medications you are on. The more medications you are taking, the harder time you will have with every other part of your body.

Along with this, above all, drink at least six glasses of water a day. Eight is preferred, but try to drink at least six eight ounce glasses of water. Good water is suggested, not tap water. I personally drink distilled water. It is processed in different ways to get rid of any bacteria and unwanted minerals. You will be amazed at the difference in taste between distilled water and pure spring water or tap water. I buy my water in gallon jugs and drink water wherever I am going.

Be sure to urinate a lot. Your urine should definitely be clean and pure. The body parts that we are talking about are nothing but a plumbing system. That plumbing system has got to be clean. When the plumbing system in your house becomes clogged, it is only because you are putting bad stuff into it. Treat your body right and use the good Draino to flush out your system.

MEMORY

I find memory to be another interesting aspect of health because everyone, including me, has had memory problems at some point. Memory seems to fail us at times. Here are a few things that may be beneficial to your short-term memory. If your short-term memory could use a perk-up, there are two quick fixes that will surprise you by how fast and how well they work. The first one is ribonucleic acid (RNA), a little-known cousin to the vitamin B family. It's a key factor in the recall process, especially short-term memory. You can find it in most health food stores.

How much do you need? Well, Dr. George Goodheart, a doctor who does a lot of research with memory and the brain, has devised an easy test to determine how much extra RNA you may need. Stand on one foot with your eyes closed. Have a friend time you to see how many seconds you can do this. People deficient in RNA can only last a short time. Next, chew one RNA tablet and try the test again. If you see little or no improvement in your time, chew another tablet and retest yourself. The number of tablets it takes to see a significant improvement is how much your daily dose should be. Recheck days later to adjust your dosage downward as your short- term memory improves.

The second quick fix pertains to how your brain cells talk to each other through a chemical called acetylcholine, an important neurotransmitter. When it runs low, brain functions weaken the body. Studies show that taking lecithin supplements increases acetylcholine levels in the brain and improves mental abilities, particularly memory. Lecithin will provide you with acetylcholine and inositol. Inositol is another memory enhancer. In medical studies, when a group of seniors took lecithin, they exhibited fewer memory lapses and noticeably better recall. Another study involving college students found that high doses of lecithin significantly improved short-term memory and test scores. The effect occurred almost immediately. Lecithin can be purchased in capsules, liquid, or as granules. Granules are by far the least expensive form.

These reports are all substantiated by many doctors in the scientific world. As I mentioned before, I am not a doctor but a nutritional counselor and a certified hypnotherapist. I now have less short-term problems because of these particular products I have mentioned. Keep in mind that these products only work if they are taken over a period of time. Don't expect immediate results because it doesn't always happen that way.

I would like to next turn to discussing ways to sharpen the mind. Doing different types of work and learning different things help to strengthen your mind and give it new dimension. The majority of older people can expect changes in their brain and memory function, but this doesn't mean losing their faculties. Older people often take longer to learn things and also have more trouble remembering, especially when they are tired or under stress. To counter this, you should try to remember things that need to be taken care of instead of writing them down. See if you can keep that memory box open all the time. There are older people who think they are forgetting things more easily, but the reality is that they are not learning them well in the first place. Names and phone numbers are some of the most difficult things to learn and remember because they tend to be entirely arbitrary.

To improve your memory, repeat pieces of information that help concentration. Write down key information when you get it. Break up long lists of names and numbers and grocery items into separate chunks of five to seven items. Create a mental picture of yourself trying to remember. Make mental associations with the things that you want to retain. Attach a name or a word to an action or color. Stay mentally active! For example, a group of 120 high-performing individuals between the ages of seventy and eighty were tracked for ten years. Those who maintained all their mental abilities engaged in daily activities that exercised their brains. They did a lot of reading, worked on crossword puzzles, used computers, played musical instruments, and attended concerts and lectures. Without any reservation, you will feel better and sharper than you ever have before. In addition, exercising will generate more information and keep you healthier than anything else. Exercise every day if you can. If not, do something at least four times a week for one hour, including lifting weights, riding a bicycle, walking, or running.

A chemical made from Chinese moss is also important for developing a good mind. Ginkgo extracts stimulate circulation in the limbs. Some of the more distressing symptoms of bad circulation include coldness, numbness, and cramping of the limbs. In carefully controlled studies of elderly individuals, Ginkgo improved pain-free walking distances from 30% to 100%. It also corrected high cholesterol levels by 86% of classes tested. Ginkgo prevented oxygen deprivation to the heart, and it also has documented benefits in diseases of the eyes and ears, including ringing in the ears.

I have a testimonial about ringing of the ears. While working in the pharmacy, a gentleman came in who had been all over Europe trying to find a solution to ringing in his ears. He came to the pharmacy and asked if I had any ideas about how to eliminate his problem, since it was driving him insane. I asked if he had taken anything. He said he had taken a few things, mostly medications that had not done much for him. I suggested taking Ginkgo, vitamin C, and vitamin E. I suggested taking 240 to 320 mgs of Ginkgo per day. Believe or not, he came back a few days later and said the ringing in his ears had dissipated for the first time in years. He was so thankful.

Ginkgo has an incredible amount of advantages, especially in the areas I have just reiterated to you. Ginkgo extract protects against nerve toxins, both preventing and curing their effects. The extract appears to directly affect neurons, not just blood flow. As shown in a new French study, different types of extracts are being explored in Korea and elsewhere showing that water extracts are less active than those using alcohol and stronger solutions. Ginkgo is strongly recommended by many practitioners in Europe, but not so many in this country, except those who are interested in alternative medicines. If you are interested, you may want to get in touch with my people here in nutrition or talk to an herbal expert who knows a lot more about Ginkgo and can give you some ideas about how you should take it. If you are taking other prescriptions, be sure that you consult your doctor first. Gingko is not good for people who have heart problems or who are taking blood-thinning medicines. Ginkgo can thin your blood, similar to some of the doctor-recommended medications like Coumadin and things of that nature. However, in any other circumstance, it's an incredibly good herb, and I suggest you try it.

I would have to say that Ginkgo is best because it maintains blood flow to the retina. Ginkgo extracts have already been shown to inhibit deteriorating vision in the elderly. It also improves memory, brain function, cerebral circulation, peripheral circulation, oxygenation, and blood flow, while decreasing dizziness and depression. It is good for tendonitis, asthma, Alzheimer's disease, and heart diseases. Give it a try! You'll like it. Ginkgo has been sold in Europe to prevent Alzheimer's for over eighty years.

THYROID

I now want to brief you on the thyroid. The thyroid gland in our body does some wonderful things when it is healthy. It keeps our body afloat in every capacity: energy levels, sight, hearing, you name it. Every particle of your body is controlled in some degree by your thyroid. When I worked at the pharmacy, there must have been at least fifteen or twenty different variations and strengths of thyroid medication. Some people who came in actually had their thyroids removed. I don't know whether you realize it or not, but most of the products created for thyroid treatment (except for those taken for thyroid cancer) come from kelp, which comes from the sea. Iodine is found in kelp, and that is what they treat it with. You can get it at a health food store. Kelp is something that you might want to consider and see if it makes your thyroid work more efficiently.

All of these suggestions need to be taken into consideration with your doctor. You might rather take medication of a synthetic nature. I prefer to use all-natural methods. You can buy real kelp in a dry form, pill form, or powdered form from any health food store. I personally take it as a preventative. I put about a quarter to half teaspoon of powder into my regular mixture of ingredients that I take in the morning. Be sure that you look into this avenue if you are bothered by your thyroid. Many of the diagnostic treatments that are done with the thyroid never seem to pick it up, so be cautious. Kelp cannot hurt if it is taken in very small amounts. Doctors claim that if you take regular amounts of iodine, which you can find at a pharmacy, and apply it to the inner part of the skin on your arm and it disappears within a two-hour period, your body is in need of kelp or iodine. I have tried it and there are times when it stays and other times when it disappears. I take it just as a precautionary measure and, like I said, a quarter or half teaspoon of kelp powder seems to work well. Take it for three or four weeks, stop for about a week, and then continue on. Again, you will want to speak with your doctor before doing so and make sure that he does not object.

ORGAN CARE

There are some simplistic approaches to making your body (including your brain, heart, lungs, prostrate, liver, pancreas, stomach, eyes, face, skin, nose, sinuses, and sex life) feel better. You should consume one tablespoon of extra virgin olive oil twice each day, once in the morning before meals and once in the evening before you retire, as well as two ounces of Aloe vera gel two to three times a day. If you have a stomach problem now, take four or five ounces of Aloe vera gel for a week or two. I guarantee you'll start feeling better. It is almost a miracle, but I have found that these things work. I take Aloe vera gel every single day and I used to have terrible problems with my stomach. I even went into the emergency room a couple of times and had the light dropped down my throat twice to look at the inside of my stomach. Doctors couldn't find anything wrong with me. Again, it's one of the reasons I spent fifty years of my life looking for alternatives. Aloe vera healed my stomach like a miracle.

For the estimated thirteen million Americans with urinary incontinence, problems with bladder control can severely disrupt daily life. Some people don't always make it to the bathroom in time, or they can't hold it in when they cough or sneeze. Some even curtail social activities because they don't have proper bladder control. Yet the majority of people with this condition never see a doctor. This is because they are either too embarrassed or they assume it is a normal part of getting older. Not true. About 80% of patients can regain nearly normal bladder control with lifestyle changes, necessary medication, or surgery.

As a bladder fills with urine, it actually sends signals to the brain that tells a person it's time to go. Before that happens, the bladder wall relaxes to permit urine to accumulate. This process is what allows most people to wait hours before going to the bathroom. Urinary control is also achieved by a ring of muscles called the urinary sphincter. It contracts to hold urine and relaxes to let it out. This action is called a Kegel. Kegel is an exercise that you can do by putting pressure into the anal area, holding momentarily, and then pushing forward into the urinary area. These can be done by a man or woman. A man does it with his penis and woman with her uterine area.

Incontinence occurs when there is a problem with either the muscular or nervous system control or a combination of both. Women are about twice as likely as men to have incontinence, although men who have prostate enlargement or prostate surgery have an increased risk of incontinence. Stress incontinence is the most common, affecting at least 50% of the woman who have urinary incontinence. It occurs when the urinary sphincter is not strong enough to hold in urine, particularly during activities that cause an increase in abdominal pressure. These include laughing, coughing, sneezing, and even exercise. Stress incontinence usually occurs during pregnancy and can persist in a woman who has had several vaginal births. Large babies and long labors can stretch and weaken the pelvic floor muscles and/or damage some of the bladder nerves. The drop in estrogen that occurs after menopause can weaken the urethra, inhibiting its ability to hold back the flow of urine.

Urge incontinence often is caused by inflammation or irritation to the bladder or urethra due to infection. This causes frequent and sudden urges to urinate. This type of incontinence may be caused by bowel problems and neurological problems, such as stroke or Parkinson's disease.

There is also overflow incontinence. Patients with nerve damage due to diabetes, for example, consistently dribble urine because they are unable to empty the bladder completely after urinating. Other potential causes of incontinence are an enlarged prostate gland, a tumor in the urinary tract, and bladder cancer. A majority of patients have stress or urge incontinence, or a combination of both known as mixed incontinence. Most types of incontinence can be diagnosed with medical history alone. Keep a bladder diary for a week or two before you see a doctor and write down how often you urinate, when you leak, and if you have trouble emptying your bladder. The answers to these questions are usually sufficient for a definite diagnosis.

We talked a little earlier about Kegel exercises. Patients are advised to squeeze the same muscles they would use to stop the flow of urine. Contract the muscles for three to five seconds, relax, and then repeat again. Do this cycle several times daily, working up to more reps each time. Kegels are helpful for both stress and urge incontinence cases. Kegels are the secret to eliminating a lot of these problems. There are drugs that doctors usually prescribe to help, but there are usually many side effects. My suggestion for urinary incontinence and things of this nature can be helped with multiple vitamins, such as C and E, and many others that do a tremendous job for the urinary tract. Drinking a lot of water and different forms of fruit juices helps immensely. In addition, eliminating a lot of stress helps as well.

Remember one thing when any form of obstruction becomes obvious in a part of the body: Blood flow is crucial to that certain area. Increased blood flow can increase the possibility of healing. There are many different forms of exercises in which you can partake. Sometimes running is not the best. Suggested activities are weight lifting, Kegels, and walking, especially for women. Doing exercises such as these helps you much more than just taking some form of medication. Please exercise and take supplements that work. Use omega-3 fatty acids. Consume a tablespoon of extra virgin olive oil every day for a week or two. You'll see a tremendous amount of changes with just these simple examples. God bless and I hope this works because it has worked for me in the past. I have noticed that if I am stressed out for any reason, these techniques help to settle my bladder.

INFLAMMATION

I would like to discuss how to reduce the pain of arthritis without the use of anti-inflammatory medications. If you do have arthritis, you have probably tried painkillers and heating pads. You may have even tried drugs like Celebrex or supplements like glucosamine. But there are five little-known remedies that you probably haven't tried. They are safe, inexpensive, and can probably curb some of the symptoms dramatically.

The first remedy is to drink green tea. Research shows that green tea is rich in polyphenols. These kinds of compounds suppress the expression of the key gene involved in arthritis inflammation. Black tea is made of the same leaves and may be just as beneficial even though it is processed differently. Drink one or two cups. Also, you should try to drink it without any caffeine.

Second, be sure to look into the most essential vitamins you can ever put in your body—vitamins C and D. These are believed to slow the loss of cartilage due to osteoporosis or osteoarthritis.

While a diet low in vitamin D has been shown to actually speed the progression of osteoarthritis, in recent high-profile studies, doctors discovered that patients who ate a diet rich in vitamin D or who took vitamin D supplements reduced their risk for worsening their arthritis by as much as 75%. Another study of over 25,000 people with a low intake of vitamin C showed that this could increase their risk of developing arthritis. Take daily supplements that provide 1,000 to 5,000 mgs of vitamin C and 400 IU of vitamin D. This is recommended by science. I personally recommend that everyone take at least 3,000 mgs of vitamin C a day. In a worsening situation, such as the onset of a cold or the flu, you can take up to 10,000 mgs.

I read an article that was written not too long ago about a doctor named Linus Pauling, whom I mentioned previously. He died when he was around ninety-five years old. During his life, he took as much as 19,000 mgs of vitamin C. He strongly believed in it and claimed that it prevented many maladies. He indicated over and over that vitamin C could prevent breast cancer, prostate cancer, and many other forms of cancer. He found that vitamin C reduces the severity of colds and the flu.

Also, you may want to try willow bark or boswellia. Willow bark is where aspirin comes from. Boswellia has been used for centuries to reduce inflammation and maintain healthy joints. A study showed that taking these two herbs is just as effective as taking a drug like Motrin. Take 240 mgs of willow bark and 1,000 mgs of Boswellia each day.

Another healthy ingredient that everyone knows about is a wonderful fruit that has been a part of life since the beginning. Eating grapes is an excellent way of decreasing your progression of arthritis and suppressing inflammation. Grape skins contain a natural compound called resveratrol. This chemical both suppresses and deactivates the enzyme that produces inflammation at the site of injury or pain. A study published in the *Journal of Biological Chemistry* confirmed that resveratrol acts as an antioxidant. Eat one cup of grapes, white or red, daily. The good news is that purple grape juice and wine also contain resveratrol. Wine is beneficial to your health, and the alcoholic content also makes you feel pretty good—but drink with reservation.

THERAPEUTIC TAPING

Therapeutic taping is wrapping tape around a joint to realign support and take pressure off. It has great benefits for arthritis sufferers. In an Australian study, 73% of patients with osteoarthritis experienced substantially reduced symptoms within just three weeks of therapeutic taping. The benefits were comparable with those achieved using standard drug treatments, and lasted even after taping was stopped. It is important to remember that taping must be done properly to be effective. You should consult a physician or a physical therapist about this— preferably a physical therapist who might be more knowledgeable about what needs to be done in comparison to a medical doctor. That particular practitioner can help show you or a family member the proper technique.

These are some of the ways in which we as practitioners use herbs and other methods to reduce the pain and suffering of a human being. We need all the help we can get. The above may be extremely good advice through which you can get reasonable or great healing. Forgive me for skipping around to various parts of the body, but I have a lot of information to give you.

ALLERGIES

Now let's talk about allergies and how they affect different people. Like everything else in this book, I have personal experience with allergies. I wake up each and every morning sneezing, and I have a runny nose that continues to bother me. My sinuses get infected. I have been to ear, nose, and throat doctors many times who charge an enormous amount of money to check you out. They gave me drugs to take that usually did not agree with me. I have found out that many people become immune to a drug naturally and also experience other side effects, such as drowsiness. Antihistamines, and various other commodities, cause many different types of problems for different people.

Sometimes when I wake up in the morning I even blow fragments of blood out of my nose, which can be caused by inflammation or dryness in the air. Low humidity can irritate your nostrils and sinuses. Most significantly, sinus problems and allergies will cause mucus to run down your throat. They shatter your vision to a degree, and stop up your ears. Sinus problems and allergies do many things that cause physical problems. This wears you down because of all the mucus that comes down from your sinuses. Living in an area where the environment is more detrimental than others, like in Missouri for example where the mold count is high, can add to the problem. People who have hay fevers maybe have them on a seasonal basis, but I, unfortunately, have them twenty-four-seven. I have to doctor these fevers in my own way as I have done with other things in my life. I find that I get the most significant results when I do so the natural way.

I have tried to find a natural cure for allergies. The natural way to help allergies, in my opinion, is by using a saline solution, which is a mixture of baking soda and salt. A quarter of the mixture is baking soda and three-quarters of it is salt, preferably sea salt. I make the mixture in a couple of different quantities, but for one quantity, mix one-fourth teaspoon of baking soda with one-half teaspoon of sea salt. Put this in an atomizer or a container. Add four ounces of water and mix. Using a dropper, take one drop of the solution and bend your head over between your knees. Let the solution run into your sinuses on each side. I take three or four droppers full in each nostril and hold my head between my knees for a period of a minute to a minute and a half. Then I take my fingers and hold my nostrils with my forefinger and my thumb, after which I release and dump the remaining solution from my nose into the sink. Then I blow out my nose on each side, but I don't blow too hard because it could hurt my ears. This is a treatment that I do when I am in significant pain. Many of the patients to whom I have suggested it all say that it has helped immensely.

A quick note: When you make the mixture, preferably use distilled water because it has no minerals in it and will not affect your sinuses in any way. Do not, and I repeat, DO NOT, use tap water. In my opinion, it is full of contaminants and is too filthy to drink. Either utilize it in a boiled condition or buy distilled water.

Allergies can be caused by many things, as you are probably aware. Sometimes they can be caused by things within the confines of your own home. Often times, people have allergies to food. I've dealt with food allergies for as long as I can remember. I remember one time when I went to an allergist who did ninety blood samples and found an enormous amount of things that I was allergic to. They included fruits and vegetables of all magnitudes, and also grains. What I found out, believe it or not, is something that everyone should take a look at when you considering allergies.

What is it that we consume every day, probably in large amounts, and pay no attention to? It is wheat. I found out I was allergic to wheat, barley, rye, and so many other grains. I had to change my eating habits. I was not allergic to rice, so I started to use a lot of rice products, which included me cooking my own brown rice. I prefer that most people eat brown rice because it has more nutrients and bioflavonoids than white rice and is also excellent for your health. It has a lot of carbohydrates in it, but you do not have to eat it every day. You can buy rice bread and many other things at health food stores. Unfortunately, this can be expensive. I have to say to myself, "Am I worth it?" The always seemingly answer, "Yes, I am tired of feeling bad."

You need to respect your body and pay attention to what you are eating. Most people don't take food allergies into great consideration. But allergies are your body's way of telling you at times what is good and bad for you. When you eat something and you don't feel good, isn't it natural to say, "Hey, my body doesn't like this." So we must take this into consideration.

I suggest taking echinacea to help your allergies. I take three echinacea three times a day when I have an uncontrollable runny nose, watery eyes, etc. In addition, I also take vitamins C and E. When my allergies are bad, I take as much as 6,000 to 7,000 mgs of vitamin C per day, but not all at one time. Also, I take nettles, which do many things for your immune system, as does echinacea. These particular products are essential when you are having problems with your sinuses. If you're not in control of all of your allergies, you'll have no way of knowing what is causing your problems. You can become downright sick because of allergies. So watch your food, and *do not* consume processed foods.

I think I can hear all of the readers who have had problems saying, "I'm not going through all this trouble to get better. I'll just go to the doctor and he'll give me a pill." That is what most people do, and this is what I am totally against. I think all doctors supply all the wrong medicines. Perhaps the medicines aren't wrong, but they just have so many side effects. What you might not realize or take into consideration is that almost all doctors only know what they were taught in medical school. If you are going to see a practitioner, see one who has the ability to prescribe some of the non-prescription supplements that they know will work. The practitioners who study alternative methods have found what a wonderful treatment these can be for their patients.

SINUSES

I'd like to talk next about a couple of things that work well for sinuses—things that work wonders for people who have sinus problems and can't seem to find anything that works. Some over-the-counter drugs don't always work and have side effects. Stinging nettles do many wonders to help relieve congestion and mucus. They're an immune builder that helps the mucous membranes of your sinuses. I take 500 mg doses twice a day when my sinuses are giving me more of a problem than normal.

I've had allergies all my life, and some foods that I eat seem to magnify the problem. Smoking, of course, is detrimental to your health and will definitely upset your sinuses. When you are in need of something you've never heard mentioned before, try nettles.

Now I want to go back to what was mentioned in the beginning of this book. If you find life extremely complicated in regards to your health, your wellbeing, and all of the other things that make you feel you're not the person you would like to be, that's what this book is all about. This book will also help relate what you can do to refurbish yourself to better health. This is a simple way in which one can understand and not have to follow all the dogma of many other books that are out there on health. This book contains simple language coming from a simple man who has worked at this for almost fifty years, trying to unravel the problems and complications that come with life. I have been there and know what I'm talking about. I hope that this will help you gain confidence in your ability to service the predicaments in your life.

PAIN

All of us experience pain many times in our lives from various causes. It can be serious (chronic), or it could be just a passer. But in all reality, there are things out there that help pain immensely. Some ingredients that can give a tremendous amount of relief are flax seed oil, borage oil, salmon oil, and cod liver oil. They can help to turn off the pain. So can wild ginger and cinnamon. These things sound so ridiculously inadequate or passé that most people pass them up because they believe only the doctors have the cure for pain. When you have severe pain such as postoperative pain or a broken bone, there are alternative things out there that can relieve it. However, you ultimately want to get the energy flowing through your body that will help you heal and cause the pain to subside.

The pain reliever that I witnessed being prescribed most when I worked in the pharmacy was called Percocet. It is a prescription drug and a controlled substance. You don't want to take these kinds of drugs if you don't have to. Whenever possible, you want to find a natural solution. As far as the Chinese are concerned, they feel that when there is pain, there isn't enough energy flow. For headache pain, there are herbs such as feverview, canine, and valerian, and thiamin and amino acids are found in the leaves of green tea.

Many of these things help immensely, but my primary objective here is to talk about the oils that do a great job. I have been taking oils for many years. For example, I mentioned that I take extra virgin olive oil. It is so easy, yet most people won't take it because they think it is too simplistic. Yet it helps relieve and prevent pain. I take two tablespoons of it a day. It also helps with relieving or preventing constipation and puts a glow into your skin that you wouldn't believe. It's just beautiful. Olive oil has vitamin E, and it helps prevent heart problems.

Many people take cod liver oil. It's a biblical thing. If you're into God, as I am, you will know that there were many biblical healings in the time of Christ. Olive oil was one of them, so you might want to give it a shot in regards to pain. But along with olive oil, flax seed oil, borage oil, cod liver oil, salmon oil, and other oils of this nature do a tremendous job for prevention. Most people my age have an enormous amount of pain. I basically don't have any pain.

Another idea is to drink an eight ounce glass of grape juice without sugar, additives, or preservatives. You can get that, and a lot of the other products I've mentioned, at the market. It is good to drink eight ounces twice a day, including once in the morning and once in the evening. This does a great job relieving pain and it has a tremendous amount of antioxidants. Of course the A's, B's, and C's that you can get from a multivitamin are great. This, too, can help people with pain.

I have mentioned to you that I am a certified hypnotherapist. We treat pain, but only with a prescription from a doctor because this is the law. Many people who are hypnotized are relieved of pain that they have had for many years. These are just areas that you may want to pursue. Another is acupuncture. I believe very strongly in acupuncture. I personally have had things in my life that I couldn't get rid of, and finally I had them cured through acupuncture. I started feeling like new. All of these things are great and are done naturally without all of the side effects of prescription drugs.

There are many other pain busters out there. Pain is an indicator that there is something bothering a part of your body. God put blood in our bodies. That is the purification of everything in our body, and when we have a lack of blood flow in an area of our body, we are going to feel a certain discomfort. Circulation is promoted with many other forms of vitamin E, vitamin C, and exercise. Exercise is so important because it releases endorphins and promotes the release of natural cortisone. There are methods of deep breathing that are very effective. There are so many things that we could talk about forever.

People who are overweight and have a poor diet are often more prone to pain. Fatty tissue is an endocrine-producing organ. Studies show that patients who are overweight release high levels of cytokines, reactive protein, and other pro-inflammatory chemicals, which are substances that promote joint and tissue damage and increase pain. The good news is that losing as little as ten pounds can significantly reduce inflammation, pain, and stiffness, regardless of the underlying cause of discomfort. People who combine weight loss with a diet that includes anti-inflammatory foods and excludes pro-inflammatory ones can reduce pain up to 90%. That rivals the effects of ibuprofen and similar painkillers without the side effects of gastrointestinal upset, etc. This in itself is very helpful because most people on diets usually have gastrointestinal upset.

Particular saturated fats need to be eliminated if you are seriously trying to free yourself of pain. The saturated fat in beef, pork, lamb, and other meats are among the main causes of painful inflammation. People who eat a lot of meat, including poultry, consume arachidonic acid. This is a fatty acid that is converted into an inflammatory chemical in the body. Although a vegetarian diet is ideal for reducing inflammation and promoting weight loss (no more than 6% of vegetarians are obese), few Americans are willing to give up meat altogether. Therefore, I recommend a plant-based diet that includes no meat or poultry and at least two to four servings of fish, fiber, and anti-inflammatory foods a week. Patients who follow this diet and limit their daily calories to about 1,400 can lose anywhere from ten to twenty-five excess pounds within three months.

It takes at least two to three weeks to establish a new dietary habit. People who give up meat entirely usually find that they don't miss it after a few weeks. Those who continue to eat some meat may find the cravings harder to resist. These are exceptional facts that have been established. There are a million diets out there and every single one of them revolves around what you eat. The scientific results of these diets are proven facts, so they subsequently have some positive effects on the body. I have never been overweight and I have eaten meat periodically. Meat is not one of my favorites, and I eat more fish than I do meat. If I do eat meat, it is usually a meat that has very little fat in it, such as a good steak.

HORMONES

I want to touch a little bit on hormones and how they affect our aging process. There are many questions about the use of hormones, such as how do hormones work within each and every one of us, how do they affect our entire lives, and how do they affect our brain and every critical organ in our body and our blood vessels?

Hormones are essential. They are a part of our entire body, and as we age, they seem to slow down manufacturing themselves. Anyone over forty years of age can honestly say their hormones are dissipating. This is not true with everyone, but for the most part, it is. Anyone over thirty-five or forty starts to have declining hormones, develops minor health ailments, and experiences a noticeable loss in his/her sense of wellbeing. Our desires and vitality can deteriorate rapidly unless we take some aggressive steps to restore the biochemistry to its youthful profile. Some chemicals that help are the adrenaline in our body, the human growth hormone, and a dozen others.

Dehydroepiandrosterone, or DHEA, produces many helpful attributes to our immune system. When you buy it at the store, it is labeled with the abbreviation DHEA, and the reference to dehydroepiandrosterone is at the bottom. This hormone is deficient in almost everyone over the age of thirty-five. A wealth of data has been collected about it for many years. Some of the problems associated with its deficiencies include chronic inflammation, immune dysfunction, depression, rheumatoid arthritis, Type 2 diabetic complications, greater risk of certain cancers, excessive body fat, cognitive decline, heart disease in men, and osteoporosis.

The good news is that DHEA has a replacement therapy. I currently take it. There was a time when I stopped taking DHEA for a while. I was feeling pretty good and ran out of the supply, so I decided to go off of it. Recently I started back up again because my vitality seemed to be depleting a little bit and I needed something to pick it up. Once again, I'd like to remind all my beautiful readers that I have personal experience with this treatment and I wouldn't recommend it otherwise. I have suggested DHEA to my clients, and those who take it seem to get a great deal of benefit from it.

DHEA, when it comes to chronic inflammation, seemingly has some inflammatory chemicals known as cytokines that increase with age and contribute to some of the degenerative diseases, such as rheumatoid arthritis and autoimmune disorders. The lesser amount of cytokines we have, the more we are exposed to certain diseases. Androgens and male hormones generally appear to be protective against the development of autoimmune diseases. As an important precursor to various androgens, DHEA has many anti-aging properties. This is where I really shine. Research shows that DHEA improves neurological function, memory, mood, and helps alleviate stress disorders. This information about DHEA comes from a study of people taking 50 mgs a day of DHEA over a six-month period that showed how DHEA restored youthful serum levels of hormones to both men and women. Men taking 100 mgs a day of the hormone reported an increase in lean body mass and muscle strength, although this does appear to be excessive in women. Any time you take hormones, you want to get approval from your doctor. Some doctors will say yes, while others will say no, so give it a shot. I personally take 25 mgs of DHEA twice a day.

DHEA has also been shown to significantly elevate the insulin growth factor (IGF). The reason this is important is because aging causes a decline in IGF levels that contribute to the loss of lean body mass and excess fat accumulation. It can cause neurological impairment and age-related immune dysfunction. Some DHEA proponents point to studies showing that this hormone protects against arteriosclerosis and heart diseases. Others show that DHEA inhibits abnormal blood platelet aggregation, a factor in sudden heart attack and stroke. DHEA adds to brain power by helping to release a product called acetylcholine, which has to do with lecithin productivity of the brain. This is needed for learning and halting memory declines. DHEA increases the acetylcholine, which helps the neurotransmitters related to lecithin that come from the gut into the brain. Lecithin creates inositol and choline, which are great brain improvers.

There has been research about using DHEA to prevent Alzheimer's disease. Studies usually find an increase in levels of the stress hormone cortisol and lower DHEA in patients with Alzheimer's disease. We know for sure that excess cortisol damages the hippocampus and is associated with the formation of plaque, an abnormal structure that is one of the hallmarks of Alzheimer's disease. If you are over thirty-five, you might want to consider the introduction of DHEA supplements.

There is another benefit of DHEA that I've researched quite a bit: life extension. Take it for a period of six months to see what kind of results you get. Then, if the results are satisfactory, you can reduce the amount of your intake. You should consult your doctor and make sure he gives you the go ahead. Take DHEA into consideration. I think it holds great possibilities for your health and anti-aging program.

SEX

In this segment, I want to talk a little bit about sex. I still enjoy it! I think sex, without any question, is a beautiful thing. God made sex for the purpose of a man and a woman to have children. He wanted to populate the entire earth with our species.

Sex gives satisfaction and also releases tension. I have not and do not use any form of chemicals for sex, like the prescription drugs Viagra or Cialis. For those of you who have different diseases, it is understandable why your sexual desires may have depleted. There are ways, with the permission of your doctors, to naturally have a better sex life. There are some amino acids that a person can take. One of them happens to be the amino acid L-arginine, which decreases blood pressure. L-arginine has been around forever and is one of the twelve or fourteen different forms of amino acids that have been documented and researched for many years. It aids sexual desire and helps men have an erection in a normal, natural way. It also reduces high blood pressure for those of you who are taking drugs for blood pressure. Erectile dysfunction and high blood pressure medications are noted to have this effect.

Working in the pharmacy, I found that those who were taking prescription drugs were always suffering from erectile dysfunction. Women's desire had become suppressed at times as well. People who have diabetic diseases, heart trouble, and many forms of health problems are certainly going to experience some of these sexual problems.

Some care-free sex is causing many health problems. Those problems, as you know, are diseases in the venereal area and HIV, which is so wide-spread and common today. There is always need for protection. Sex must be with someone you care about. This will increase your desire, and you can have a much better sex life if you are healthy. Along with L-arginine, I suggest taking Ginkgo. Remember that the consumption of alcoholic beverages depletes your sex drive because it constricts the blood flow in your arteries. That's why I suggest taking Ginkgo and L-arginine. You can take up to 1,500 mgs of L-arginine without problems, and like everything else, some of it can be taken in excess. Here again, you need to discuss this with your practitioner, although it works wonders for me.

These items need to be taken consistently. They do not work like Viagra, Cialis, or some of the other mood-enhancing drugs created for instant gratification. L-arginine and Ginkgo need to be taken at least thirty days before you see a difference. Talk to your practitioner about it. These two items have no known side effects. I've been taking them for years, and others who have taken these alternative prescriptions highly recommend it.

To enhance your primary relationship, you can schedule special time with your spouse or partner. Develop joint activities and be sure to communicate. Even better, make a conscious decision to do something on a regular basis, such as buying flowers or writing a loving letter. Psychologists have found that this sort of behavior causes your attitude toward the other person to become more caring and automatic. Aim toward more satisfying sex. Even at my age, I have all the desire and good health to make sex a good, satisfying activity. Sex is a beautiful part of life and there are some people who have lost their desire completely. This is why men are taking Viagra and many other substances to improve their sex life. Their sex life is poor because they have deficiencies throughout their entire body, which causes erectile dissatisfaction.

I want to create a special section in regard to sex and the satisfaction that goes with it. People lose a lot in life to satisfy their partner, and sex is definitely involved. The most important thing of all is to have a loving relationship. In the end, this means good sex. One-night stands and quickies, in my humble opinion, just don't seem to give you the satisfaction you are looking for. Here I am in my eighties and I still have a fantastic sexual desire because my health is excellent. You must do what's right physically and mentally. The mind, body, and spirit create a synergy that does more than you could possibly imagine. When you have these three ingredients working together to maintain the goodness of life, sex comes into play. Even if you do not have a partner, the desire is there because God has put that desire into your mind and there is nothing wrong with it.

Sex is a God-given privilege, but it has been abused in many ways, and I don't think I need to elaborate on how it's been abused. Sometimes people use sex in an abnormal way, and this causes a lot of problems. You know the type of prevention you must use. If not, you need to see a special counselor to find out. It is well publicized in schools and all over the world. There are too many diseases involved with abnormal sex, so pick and choose your partners wisely.

I have a tendency to sometimes repeat myself when I'm talking about different forms of nutrition, but I want to give you the best advice I can. My children have strongly encouraged me to write this book so others can learn what I've discovered throughout my life. I worked in a pharmacy for eleven years, and for every person who came in there who was taking drugs, whether for their heart, high blood pressure, cholesterol, you name it, there were just thousands of different forms of medications that were prescribed depending on the type of physician. Even though I wasn't allowed, I did some research on these people and found out that their sex desire had gone down. When this happens, the physician puts you on Viagra, Cialis, or another medication that enhances the sex drive. Then you have to worry about how long the erection will last.

This is not the way you want to do it. I've tried an alternative and I know it works. The amino acid L-arginine has many of the same ingredients found in Viagra and all of the other sexual dysfunction medications. You can take up to 1,500 mgs of L-arginine each day. You'll begin to notice its effects after two to three weeks. If sex is on your mind, you don't have to take medications to help you have an erection. There is a healthy normal way. It works wonders for most people. If you have had prostate cancer or some other problems, I'm not sure if it will work. But I do know one thing—it certainly won't hurt to try it. Doctors won't prescribe these alternative medications because they usually don't know anything about them, or they haven't been trained that way. It is something you might want to try if you have sexual problems or want to prevent prostate problems. You can take it with lycopene and all of the other supplementations I have been talking about. Good luck. I am sure it will work if you try it. Always give God a word or two and ask him for his help.

THE ESSENTIALS

To prevent allergies or any other problems that may be bothering you, look into the supplements that contain vitamins A, C, E, all the B complexes, and selenium. I already mentioned the recommended doses of these products. You should take beta-carotene, the precursor to vitamin A, because too much vitamin A can cause jaundice. You can take up to 25,000 IU of beta-carotene. If you are having severe problems, you might take up to 50,000 IU, as well as all of the B complexes. I would prefer to take B complex 100, which contains the seven different forms of vitamin B that are essential to you, including B12, and gives you 100 mgs in each of these departments. Vitamin C can be taken at 3,000 mgs per day on a normal basis. For vitamin E, I would suggest 400 to 800 IU daily. I would start off at 400 IU a day for two or three months and then increase it to 800 IU. For selenium, you should take a tablet of 200 mcg.

Once again, you should eat a healthy diet. It is good to get at least seven to eight hours of sleep every night. That is crucial for your health, your eyes, and your entire body. Take a multivitamin, and be sure that it includes vitamins C and E. Those are powerful antioxidants. Use lutein, which is a carotenoid. It protects the retinal part of your eyes. Also take the amino acid called taurine. Along with selenium, magnesium, and bioflavonoids, take your fish oil capsules. Exercise aerobically. Take a break every day for fifteen minutes and rest your eyes. Practice deep rhythmic breathing. For those who have problems with their lungs and heart, deep breathing can revitalize you.

After a couple of weeks, you'll be amazed with the results. Get a regular eye exam. I think your eyes are very important, and if they are not functioning properly, exercise and supplements will help you maintain good eyesight.

SECTION 2
FOODS

OVERVIEW

You definitely want to keep track of what you are putting into your body. Never forget that food is the essential way to get ingredients into your system. Good food is what we are talking about. However, most of us do not get all the nutrition we need because we do not consume as many healthy foods as we should. Some nutritionists say that you should eat eight to ten servings of fruit a day. Well, if I did that, I'd be on the toilet all day long because fruit gives me diarrhea. I'm lucky if I can eat fruit twice a day. It's good to empty out your bowels, but too much is too much, and I don't know if I agree with the recommended servings. However, there's nothing wrong with them if you can handle them.

ALCOHOL

Moderate alcohol intake is defined as no more than two drinks a day for a man and one for a woman. Why the difference?

Well, women end up with a higher blood level of alcohol and thus become more intoxicated than men. One reason is that women tend to be smaller than men and proportionately have less fat tissue. Another reason is that the stomach enzymes that break down alcohol before it reaches the bloodstream are less active in women. Women are more likely to develop damage to the liver, heart muscles, and brain, even with lower levels of alcohol intake. Alcohol can increase a woman's risk of getting osteoporosis and breast cancer. Though women are less likely than men to drive after drinking, they have a higher risk of having fatal crashes because of their blood alcohol concentrations. Pregnant women who drink really risk the health of their babies with fetal alcohol syndrome. No level of alcohol consumption in pregnancy is known to be safe.

Don't forget your dark wine during the course of the day. The FDA says that a little wine each day is excellent for your health. Wine can give you an adequate amount of antioxidants, which ward off the free radical carcinogens that cause our blood cells to deteriorate. Make sure you get a little bit of this good wine. Even back in biblical days, Jesus Christ and his disciples frequently drank wine, so there must be something to it. Give it a try. I have wine every day. It appears that some people can handle wine better than other alcoholic beverages. Just remember that none of the other alcoholic beverages consumed have the antioxidants that wine delivers, especially red wine.

BERRIES

There are a number of extensively researched foods out there that I think you should know about. One of them happens to be the blueberry. When I was in the military, we would eat blueberry jam before we would take any night flights, which helped to sharpen our nighttime vision and make everything come into better focus. The blueberry is considered to be a brain-protection fruit. A leading scientist, Dr. James, once the head CEO of the USDA, the U.S. agency for research on nutrition and aging at Canton University, calls blueberries brain-power food. Moreover, a wealth of exciting research establishes that in addition to promoting brain health, this long-prized native North American fruit may have a great range of beneficial health effects.

Blueberries can be consumed fresh, frozen, canned, or from an extract. After studying approximately twenty-four varieties of fresh fruit, twenty-three vegetables, sixteen herbs and spices, and ten different nuts and dried fruits, the U.S. Department of Agriculture determined that the blueberry scored highest overall in antioxidant capacity. That is what all of us are striving for! Antioxidants free us from the free radicals that cause diseases. Separate studies showed that blueberries may help lower cholesterol, promote urinary tract health, and reduce the risk of urinary infections. Studies in Europe have documented the benefits of consuming bilberries, which are a closely related cousin to the blueberry. They're proven to halt cataract progression and protect against glaucoma.

A handful of blueberries rinsed off with cold water and put into your fruit bowl or eaten with your cereal in the morning make a good accompaniment to soy milk. I make sure to eat blueberries every single day!

My eyesight seems to be up to par. I just went to the eye doctor not too long ago and he said I have the eyesight of a twenty-five-year-old. I attribute that to taking lutein capsules and eating blueberries. Everyone who eats blueberries seems to find them very palatable. Blueberries and bilberries belong to the proanthocyanidins species of fruits, which includes more than 450 plants grown in all parts of the world. In this group, the darkest colored fruits appear to provide the best health benefits. Scientists attribute this to the compounds that give the plants their darkest pigmentation. These bioflavonoids include antigens and their precursor, both of which are calcareous scavengers of free radicals and carcinogens. Research demonstrates that blueberry consumption boosts antioxidant levels in humans. Many helpful things come from fruits and vegetables, but blueberries seem to be at the top of the list in helping to reduce the risk of many chronic and degenerative diseases.

Studies on this beautiful little fruit keep purporting blueberries' ability to reduce lipid peroxidation, a contributor to cardiovascular disease. They are also said to suppress the growth of several types of cancer cells. That's a big item—suggesting that blueberries will play a future role in human cancer research. Incidentally, you don't need to eat blueberries all day long. A good handful rinsed off with pure water will do.

In 2005, in an article in the *Journal of Neurobiology of Aging*, Dr. James noted this fruit for its neural prospects. I found it interesting to note that this particular compound sharply reduces the problems people have with tumors. This research said that the tumors in the brain cannot metastasize with it, and that the tumors even started to diminish. This is a result of eating blueberries. Proof again that eating healthy helps you to stay healthy. No one will argue with that statement.

No studies to date have compared the effectiveness of fresh blueberries versus frozen blueberries, canned berries, or berry extracts. Each form of the fruit has been shown to contain essential anthocyanins and proanthocyanins. That makes blueberries one of the most exciting nutriceuticals being researched and consumed today. Blueberry extracts have the advantage of delivering the fruit's phytochemicals in a simple standardized dose. Regardless of how they are consumed, blueberries should be considered a mainstay of every healthy diet. This remarkable fruit has been known for centuries for its medicinal properties and continues to prove itself in research laboratories around the world.

The hawthorne berry has been very beneficial to my life. It is said that hawthorne is the berry that was on Christ's throne and was applied to his head and used as a crown. The berry itself supposedly has heavy biblical cures. I have discovered this through research and my own personal experience. At one time I had heart palpitations and even had a little bit of accelerated blood pressure. I went to the doctor and he said there was nothing wrong with my heart. He gave me a medication that just knocked me on my butt. So I did some research and found a product called hawthorne berry. It helps in the management of mild forms of arterial sclerosis, angina, and arrhythmia. Hawthorne completely relieves me and actually has a healing power for the heart. It also lowers cholesterol and blood pressure. Hawthorne berries contain flavonoids and procyanidins. Standardized hawthorne products are available in capsules and extracts. You may need to take it for four or five weeks before you see any effects. I took it for about a month and found that it helped immensely. It will also assist with pain, if you have some discomfort in that area. It will also save you a lot of money. Hawthorne is usually taken at about 550 mgs three times a day. I think you will see some marvelous results.

CHOCOLATE

For many years, nutrition experts have advised people about how much fruits, vegetables, and other healthy foods their diets should contain. However, this approach has its limitations. Some manufacturers have tried to turn ordinary foods into nutriceuticals. Nutriceuticals are a form of ingredient in a lot of foods that are dedicated to being beneficial to your health. They are fortified so that they become more like drugs. Since nearly everyone loves chocolate, and because chocolate has potential health benefits, nutriceuticals have been an object of much medical discussion lately. They have gained scientific attention, and not surprisingly, the supplement industry has tried to turn chocolate into medicine. They do this by putting various cocoa compounds into a tablet and capsule form.

Is chocolate on the verge of being reclassified as a vitamin? I hardly think so. However, the healthy components in chocolate are certain phytochemicals called flavonoids. They are also found in tea, red wine, and many fruits and vegetables. Plain cocoa without added fat and sugar has an aspirin-like effect on the blood. Thus, it helps prevent clotting. Dark chocolate, which contains more flavonoids than milk chocolate, may help lower blood pressure, reduce blood cholesterol, and benefit the heart in many ways. That's only part of the story. The Mars Company, which makes the fortified chocolate bar CocoaVia, has sponsored lots of research on chocolate. It has made other companies' foundations, and the government, see chocolate as a positive nutritional supplement.

If there is any catch to this, for the chocolate-eating public, the problem is that pure chocolate is bitter and unpalatable. Some cocoa has to be mixed with sugar, milk, fat, and other additives, but turning cocoa into a candy destroys some of the phytochemicals. Then it goes into the shiny wrapper at the store. Scientific studies usually use dark chocolate with high flavonoid content, which is unlike what you buy at the candy store. Of course, chocolate candy is high in calories. It is a more reliable source of sugar and fat than of healthy flavonoids. In reality, if you eat candy and you eat chocolate, it is preferable to eat dark chocolate. It has more beneficial effects than the lighter chocolate, which has more additives. As far as taking pills to get the additive flavonoids of chocolate, I'd rather have the chocolate myself. It is more expensive if you put it into pill or capsule form, and there is not enough evidence to recommend it. There is no guarantee that these pills or capsules contain any flavonoids or any of the ingredients that are supposedly in chocolate.

Words to the wise: I have always been pro-chocolate because I like it. Sometimes I think I am a chocoholic. I don't eat it that much, but when I do eat chocolate, it is something I want and love. I could eat a ton of it, but chocolate contains caffeine, and if you have a negative response to caffeine, you should note that large quantities of chocolate can put a lot of caffeine in your system. If you have a problem with caffeine causing heart palpitations or causing your heart to beat faster, chocolate could certainly aggravate it. Therefore, chocolate lovers should be responsible for the amount they take in. You need to pay attention to how you feel after you have eaten it. I love chocolate, you love chocolate, we all love chocolate! I don't think there's anything shameful about having chocolate.

CINNAMON

Research into the benefits of cinnamon has been promising, but not totally convincing. It's been roaming around in the minds of scientists for many years. Why don't they come up with a decision? I have positive proof from the years I spent working in the pharmacy. I suggested that people with Type 2 diabetes take a quarter teaspoon of cinnamon every morning. Cinnamon has a tremendous amount of polyphenols that may help reduce blood sugar. This has been shown in a modest amount of people with Type 2 diabetes. It lowered their blood sugar by 20-30%. It is something to look into. Along with cinnamon is an herb called vanadium. You can get it at any health food store. By taking a combination of these two substances, some people have gone off insulin completely. With exercise, they did incredible things. If you have some indications of diabetes or diabetes in your family, it might be a great preventative to try.

FISH

Ignore organic labels on fish; the term "organic" is meaningless. The USDA has not set standards on seafood with regard to fish. Always look for wild fish. We know from research that farmed fish consume too much fecal matter from other fish and have too many toxins. Try to avoid any fish other than the wild fish that comes from the sea. Wild salmon has omega fatty acids, and fish like wild salmon can reduce the risk of sudden-death heart attacks. Salmon that is caught wild has less dioxin contaminants than farmed salmon. When you buy fish, look for wild fish distributed from Alaska.

Omega-3 fatty acids will help fix many of the previously mentioned problems, so don't forget your fish. Research has confirmed how important this is, and I eat a lot of wild fish because it is has RNA and DNA. These are the acids that help to give you a better mind and excellent health and balance. Anchovies can help you sleep better. New research has indicated that people who eat a certain amount of anchovies have an enormous amount of RNA and DNA and its components. Nucleic acids help with people who have sleep disorders.

Also, eat sardines at least once a week. They are loaded with nucleic acids for a youthful appearance.

GARLIC

Garlic is another substance that has an enormous effect upon our health. Its effectiveness depends upon how you use it, when you use it, and if you use it. Garlic has been scrutinized, but has been implemented as one of the most powerful herbs in existence as far back as World War I and II. Russia and countries in Europe used this product with their troops to help the wounded, keep up their immune systems, and heal pneumonia or various other diseases. Garlic has been taking care of people for thousands of years. Within the past several decades, Americans have taken an increasing interest in garlic to help relieve and even heal heart problems and other illnesses such as cancer. The ancient Greeks and Romans used these additives as decongestants and to prevent scurvy. Garlic is one of the oldest medicines in China, dating back to 2852 BC. Dr. Fou Hough, a respected medical consultant, has promoted this product for many years, discussing how it flushes out toxins and has the power to cure illnesses.

Part of garlic's healing pros comes from the fact that it is fermented. Being naturally preserved improves its natural values. Because of its acidity, garlic closely resembles the stomach's digestive juices. It is often said that both vinegar and garlic closely resemble the proper digestion nutrients that are available today. This is especially true of apple cider vinegar. It is packed with nutrition, rich in enzymes and vitamins, and helps balance your amino acids.

Two teaspoons of garlic daily supply 19-22% of the minerals essential for good health. In the right ratio, you also need vinegar's mightiest mineral called potassium. It is so essential to every living thing that without it, there is no life, says Dr. Jarvis, MD, an advocate of the health-boosting powers of potassium and rich apple cider vinegar. Potassium helps the body to regulate the heartbeat and to get rid of excess sodium. It has a big role in controlling deadly heart disease, and also eases the pain of bursitis and arthritis. Other minerals and vinegars contain potassium additives, making them more potent than they would be on their own.

Zesty garlic lowers cholesterol, thins the blood, and prevents dangerous blood clots by making blood platelets less sticky. Studies at institutions like Tufts, Cornell, Penn State, and other universities prove garlic stops heart attacks before they begin. Compounds in the aromatic herb have been found to block the bugs that cause ulcers. According to the herbalist John Hinerman, PhD, raw garlic lowers high blood sugar levels, which eases diabetes. Celebrities with one eye on the future like Kate Mulgrew from *Star Trek Voyager*, *Murphy Brown*'s Candice Bergman, and *Halloween*'s Jamie Lee Curtis all include the goodness of garlic in their meals. Action hero Harrison Ford isn't afraid to add a hefty dose of this herb to his favorite pasta dish. There are many derivatives of garlic. The form called allicin kills cold viruses, flu viruses, and the herpes viruses that cause cold sores and venereal diseases.

Studies have demonstrated garlic's ability to kill bacteria resistant to antibiotics, and meat-seasoned garlic has protected against the killer *E. coli*. Allicin and its related compounds have been found to lower bad cholesterol levels by 15%. Garlic packs a powerful anti-cancer trace element, selenium. Researchers at Cornell University and the National Cancer Institute proved that garlic significantly reduces the risk of stomach and colorectal cancer. Other studies show that garlic wipes out breast cancer in mice and wards off bladder cancer in animals. Veteran broadcaster Barbara Walters turned to garlic after researching its anti-cancer properties. "I have a family history of colon and breast cancer and it scares me, so I eat a lot of garlic and I'm going to start taking garlic pills. I have never felt better. Knock on wood, my health is good."

To take advantage of garlic's preventative powers, all you need is a clove or two a day chopped in salads, minced in sauces, or cooked in soup. If straight garlic is too aromatic for you, try equally potent odorless extracts and capsules. Garlic fights head colds and is an incredible product for your health. Give it a try. For a natural cough syrup, boil lemon thickened with honey and two or three cloves of garlic. It makes a terrific cough medicine.

GINGER

I take ginger for many of my physical concerns. If you're an athlete, as I am, your stomach may sometimes become upset. If so, you can take the herb ginger. It's very settling and a great anti-inflammatory. Ginger is fantastic for people who have lightheadedness and dizziness, and for those of us who fly and go deep-sea fishing or get sea sickness. What's great is that ginger does not cause drowsiness. I normally take two tablets, a half hour before whatever the occasion is, and repeat every three to four hours. Be cautious if you take a prescription from your doctor. Nine out of ten times the drug doctors prescribe will make you so tired that you cannot enjoy your trip. Go the natural way. If you have a sore throat, gargle with ginger two times a day. Then say goodbye to that sore throat.

OILS

Looking again into the alternatives that were mentioned in previous sections, there is one powerful alternative to antibiotics. Each and every time we visit a doctor for a virus or upper respiratory infection, we could pretty much agree that we'll leave his office with a prescription for an antibiotic. Not today! There have been reports of resistant strains of deadly bacteria that have the medical community thinking twice before dispensing antibiotics. Therefore, the public is thinking twice before taking them.

A new herbal superstar we have discussed is olive oil and extra virgin olive oil. Previously, some claimed that the olive leaf extract may be one natural alternative to antibiotics. This herb has been shown to both bolster the immune system and fight infections and other illnesses. To call olive leaf extract new is a bit misleading; the medical uses of this plant have been growing since the early 1800s when olive leaf extract was used to treat malaria.

During the past forty years, European researchers have been gradually piecing together information on the active component. The active agents of antimicrobials are a component in the olive leaf. The leaf is further broken down into a substance called elenolic acid, a powerful antiviral and antibacterial agent which is extremely safe and nontoxic. Even at high doses, elenolic acid has been shown to fight viruses and bacteria in laboratory tests. However, elenolic acid must be specially processed to render its effectiveness in the human body. After many frustrating false starts, researchers finally developed and perfected an effective production method during the early 1990s and a product known as calcium elenolate became available to clinicians. Today, neuropathic physicians and herbalists use it to treat a wide variety of infections, as well as colds, flu, hepatitis, and herpes.

In 1999, an Italian study showed that olive leaf extract was related to the compound that was effective in preventing a wide variety of respiratory bacteria, including influenza and streptococcus. In studies involving animals, it was shown to increase nitrate-oxide levels, which is an indication of improved immune response. In 1962, scientists showed that olive leaf extract would be effective in treating heart disease. Tests have shown that olive leaf works to lower blood pressure by dilating blood vessels and increasing circulation. Researchers attribute this to its oleuropin, which is also a powerful antioxidant and flavonoid that reduces LDL, or bad cholesterol. Olive leaf also contains several polyphenols. These are flavonoids, including hesperin and quercetins, which are beneficial to heart health. As if this weren't enough, still more potential medical uses exist for this panacea-like extract.

Researchers in Spain have studied diabetic rats and determined that olive leaf has an anti-diabetic quality. European physicians are also using olive leaf for healing injuries. One recent animal experiment performed in Turkey at the university demonstrated that olive leaf substantially increased the healing speed of injured tissue. It is used for preventing the flu and the common cold, and to treat high blood pressure and diabetes. This little Mediterranean fruit has proven to be a powerhouse in herbal medicine and scientists believe even more medicinal uses lie on the horizon.

Fried foods can cause migraines. To be healthy, opt more often for lower-temperature cooking methods, such as baking, boiling, steaming, or microwaving. If you fry at home, pan frying is better than deep frying. Don't put breading on your food, and reduce some of the fats by draining fried food on a paper towel. Also, try to avoid foods cooked in reused oil. You should stay away from it, so pay attention when you are in a restaurant. If a part of your meal is fried and the crust is darkened, the food was cooked in reused oil. Therefore, send it back or don't eat it. The reused oil increases your LDL which affects your cholesterol tremendously. Be wary of menu items described as battered, breaded, or crispy, and if you are unsure of something, ask your server.

Another beneficial tidbit is this: Do not forget your extra virgin olive oil. Olive oil is more stable when heated, and thus forms fewer degradation byproducts. Understand that extra virgin olive oil is tremendously good oil. The oil helps your heart and lungs. If you've got a cough you can't seem to get rid of, a tablespoon of olive oil taken internally does wonders. You cannot cook food with olive oil if it's going to require temperatures over 160 degrees. If it boils, it acts in a reverse fashion. Don't preheat oils longer than necessary, and use a vent fan when frying so that you can keep the odor and toxins out of the air.

Some people just cook with it, but I take olive oil every day. I swallow two tablespoons—one in the morning and one in the evening. It is excellent for every part of your body. It helps prevent arthritis and other inflammatory diseases.

SODIUM

You want to take a look at the sodium content of your food products. Some products that have high sodium content are tomato sauce, chicken soup, anchovies, a Big Mac, chicken pot pies, cottage cheese, sauerkraut, Canadian bacon, and vegetable juice cocktail. Olives contain the smallest amount of sodium. The highest content is tomato sauce, which contains 1,280 mgs per cup. You should try to lower your sodium intake and increase your potassium. Some foods that have a high potassium content are white beans, lima beans, spinach, lentils, sweet potatoes, halibut, oranges and orange juice, bananas, broccoli, avocados, artichokes, grapefruit, pork and beef, corn, milk, salmon, and cereal.

SOY

The next segment that I want to discuss is the joy of soy. You should take advantage of this laudable legume. It has heart-smart power. Soy comes in many variations, such as tofu, miso, edamame, soy sauce, soy milk, tempeh, and even in soy protein shakes. Few plants can match soy's widespread dietary influence. Historical references indicate that soy has been cultivated since 11 BC, but its emergence as a superstar in the United States has only been in the last two decades. The average American consumes about five grams of soy each day. Research shows that soy sales went from 8.52 million in 1992 to 3.7 billion in the year 2002. In Japan, however, the average soy intake is 55 grams per day, which in part accounts for how Japan's cardiovascular mortality rates are half those of the United States.

Evidence has linked soy to anti-cancer bone-building and menopause-mitigating properties. This little legume's main claim to fame is its ability to promote heart health. Researchers have attributed soy's heart-healthy benefits with a singular complex of isoflavonoids. These isoflavonoids are phytoestrogens, plant compounds that act like estrogen in the body. Soy's protein content further sets it apart from other plants. Soy contains complete protein possessing all the necessary amino acids to promote growth and development.

I quit drinking regular milk twenty years ago when I discovered how many additives it contains. I thought it wasn't worth it and I felt that I had some allergic resistance to milk, so I subsequently started eating and drinking soy and using tofu. You can buy it in different quantities, and as far as texture is concerned, you can buy it in whatever form you like. You can fry it in a pan and make it almost taste like meat. It's excellent with eggs in the morning. You can generate a good taste for it. I have it every day. I take the soy milk, which is organic, and I use it on my cereal. I drink vanilla-flavored soy milk. The great part is that it comes in different flavors, quantities, and sizes. If you have a special taste you like, you can certainly get it in a soy product.

Studies that were published in *The New England Journal of Medicine* in 1995 showed that soy reduces the risk of heart disease. The study, which analyzed thirty-eight clinical studies, concluded that soy protein consumption may have worked to lower cholesterol and LDL (which is the bad cholesterol) when compared with animal protein. The FDA, which is notoriously strict about approving breakthrough claims in heart health statements, says that 25 grams of soy protein a day, as part of a diet low in saturated fats and cholesterol, may reduce the risk of heart disease. After the FDA's approval, all the research has only continued to verify soy's cardiac benefits.

The 2006 *American Journal of Cardiology* analyzed forty-one randomized-control soy supplement trials. Such supplementations were found to be associated with a significant reduction in total cholesterol and the total cholesterol in triglycerides, which is a blood fat. In 2004, the *Journal of the American Medical Association* focused on soy protein in treating obesity, hypertension, high triglycerides, increased HDL (the good cholesterol), and insulin resistance of a metabolic syndrome. Your soy target can be the FDA's 25 grams a day, or you can pursue the lofty Japanese standard of 55 grams. Health food shoppers have catered to soy protein shakes at bars for their convenience and high soy content. Thanks to an increasing variety of flavors and blends, you can appease your taste buds. You can buy soy products in just about any store. Try to keep your heart happy. It's time to discover the many joys of soy.

VINEGAR

Apple cider vinegar is one healing momma, and its powers have been known for hundreds of years. It just keeps going on and on. Here are some of the things that vinegar actually can heal or improve. Apple cider vinegar has an effect on acne, bursitis, tendonitis, cold sores, coughs, dandruff, diaper rash, foot odor, headaches, head lice, heartburn, hiccups, hives, indigestion, insect stings, jock itch, oily hair, poison ivy, scars, psoriasis, shingles, sore throat, sunburn, swimmer's ear, warts, and even yeast infections. These are some of the few things that vinegar helps. Its power for relieving symptoms and healing is incredible. I am not going to give you all of the individual mixtures for each illness just mentioned. However, the simplistic mixture to cure these problems is two tablespoons of water to one tablespoon of apple cider vinegar.

I have personally used vinegar for a rash on my face, a cough, and indigestion. As far as indigestion is concerned, I suggest that you make the mixture heavier with water. Perhaps mix six ounces of water with each tablespoon of vinegar and drink it. It will work wonders for indigestion. For jock itch, be sure to mix it heavily with water and strain it first. That area is extremely sensitive, and it only takes a little bit to put that fire out. Vinegar is excellent for poison ivy, but it has never been suggested by doctors to try it. Wash the area well with soap and water before applying the vinegar and it will outdo any of the over-the-counter drugs from the store.

Vinegar has been utilized over a period of years by people who favor homeopathic remedies. Some people swear that vinegar mixed with honey and warm water will take the pain out of leg cramps. Others use vinegar to dry up cold sores. Should someone faint, vinegar is an alternative to smelling salts. The list goes on and on. Put a drop of it on your tongue and you'll know immediately what gives the tangy liquid its sour reputation. Vinegar is acidic, thanks to a high concentration of acidic acids. Form 1 bacteria feast on the fermented liquid. Acidic acid may be kind to your body, but it is an industrial strength product that can destroy photographic film. It creates a very familiar pharmaceutical product called aspirin.

Vinegar is also good for the hair. As an acid, vinegar reacts with a chemical base to produce natural H_2O (water) along with some salt when spread on the skin or used as a hair rinse. It can remove soap, shampoo, or conditioner residue. Rinsing the hair with vinegar may also ease dandruff and itchy scalp. As I mentioned, vinegar can be used as a stomach settler. Sometimes a teaspoonful of vinegar after meals might just be the ticket to prevent indigestion.

Vinegar is a coolant, spreads on skin, and evaporates quickly, providing a friendly chill that can suppress the pain of sunburn. Vinegar can counteract the inflammation that causes sunburns to itch. It's also a fungus fighter. Most fungi flourish in the warm, moist hollow of an ear canal, and this condition is known as swimmer's ear. When vinegar is mixed with equal parts of rubbing alcohol and dropped into the ear, it can fight invaders and cure the condition. Speaking of fungus, soaking your feet in vinegar is an effective treatment for athlete's foot. If you have a problem with stinky feet, it also suppresses the odor. The vinegar content gives it a nice sharp scent and can override less lovely odors.

If you've been stung by insects or jellyfish, the sting can be relieved with vinegar. It neutralizes pain, causing the substances in the skin to become slightly watered down. You can dab it on the skin with a cotton ball. Vinegar can also relieve the itching of hives. Many people use vinegar as a remedy for headaches. The traditional approach is to soak brown paper with apple cider vinegar and apply it to the forehead. You can also soak a clean cloth in vinegar and tie it around your head. We are not sure why vinegar works, but many people swear by it. For a sore throat, don't hesitate to gargle with a little warm water and vinegar.

If you are traveling, vinegar may have many other healing purposes. Different varieties were used in the Philippines, Trinidad, and the British Isles many years ago. Elsewhere, you may run across vinegars yielded by honey, potatoes, dates, nuts, and berries. The most common kinds you'll find are wine vinegar made from grapes, cider vinegar made from apples, or plain distilled white vinegar made from grain. Among today's promoters of good health, apple cider vinegar is often favored above all. Fermented apples are rich in pectin and have a type of fiber that is excellent for digestion. Apples contain malic acid, which combines with magnesium in the body to fight aches and pains.

Should you care to make your own vinegar, it's easy. Starting with cider, our wine fermentation is sped up by the addition of a dollop of vinegar to initiate the process. Jars and utensils have to be carefully sterilized to avoid contamination with unwanted bacteria. As one's skills improve, the home brewer learns to recognize the moment when the brew is done. Once bottled, capped, and stored, homemade vinegar stays good for many months. But, for home remedies, any store-bought vinegar will do.

Have good luck with vinegar. It's simplistic, inexpensive, and extremely effective. I have tried it in many areas on my children and myself and have never had a failure yet.

SECTION 3
SUPPLEMENTS AND VITAMINS

OVERVIEW

Regarding supplements, vitamins, and other forms of herbs, certain things should be mentioned. You should take each and every one of your vitamins for a period of time and add on to each one that you are taking. I personally take about forty-five different vitamins over a period of time. I don't do that every day, but almost every day. I try to take a day off, but I have a hard time taking a day off with magnesium because I lack that mineral in my body. Therefore, I take it every day. For example, I'm sure you are aware of folic acid. Taking 800 mcg is usually sufficient to help people, especially to offset birth defects for pregnant women. It is an essential supplement.

However, synthetic forms of folic acid can trigger hives, breathing problems, and itching. That is something you should be aware of. You can normally get a good amount of natural folic acid by eating green leafy vegetables. Liver and wheat nuts are full of folic acid. So if you are eating a lot of these forms of food, you are probably getting a normal amount of folic acid already.

Research has shown that folic acid, taken by both men and

women for a period of a year, prevents heart attacks by 60%. That is something to remember. These are all scientific research evaluations that have gone on for years. Many doctors will profess that they don't believe it, but it's only because they don't know any better.

I have a little list that I call "The 10 Commandments of Supplements." There is also the "Golden Rule" for strengthening your diet. If you follow these particular commandments, you certainly will be on the way to healthier living.

First Commandment: Thou shall consider dietary supplements strictly as a compliment to a healthy diet. Supplements, as you are very much aware, are meant to substitute for the things that you are not acquiring from your daily intake of food. Dietary supplements are intended to reinforce a healthy diet and not to replace one. Despite the growing amount of research that clearly demonstrates the healthy benefits of dietary supplements, no substitutes exist for food. People need its complex make-up of fiber, nutrients, and tastes.

Second Commandment: Thou shall take a multivitamin as insurance. I must suggest my multivitamin called Ad-ditions, which can be purchased on the web. This particular multivitamin has thirty-one ingredients, including 120 mgs of Ginkgo. My product has been out now for twenty years. A study conducted by the United States government surveyed 20,000 Americans and found that not one individual consumed 100% of the recommended daily allowance. Most people realize that they don't eat the way they should, so a daily multivitamin or mineral supplement is an inexpensive insurance policy. We are talking about preventatives. Just one B vitamin, with folic acid for example, can cut heart disease risks by as much as 70%. In 1995, the *Journal of the American Medical Association* reported that 400 mcg of folic acid, the amount found in almost any multivitamin, could reduce such risks of heart attacks by 70%.

Third Commandment: Thou shall not consider RDAs as law. That's a good subject point because the RDAs, over the years, have changed dramatically. The RDAs fifteen years ago, in my opinion, were too low. New research has changed the adequacy of the RDA standards. The RDA for vitamin C, for example, was only 60 mgs. On a daily basis, I take 3,000 to 4,000 mgs of vitamin C, and if I feel as though I might be coming down with something, I increase it to as much as 10,000 mgs. Recent data suggests that 200 mgs is a more optimal intake. Vitamins A and D and some minerals are the only nutrients with RDA standards that agree with the government's study-supported optimal need. The fat-soluble vitamins A and E, as well as most minerals, should never be taken in high amounts.

The most clear-cut example of adequacy is the case of vitamin E. In 1993, the *New England Journal of Medicine* documented three well-conducted human studies that demonstrated that 100 IU of supplemental vitamin E were much more optimal than the RDA of just 30 IU, which to me is like spitting in the ocean. The average American typically ingests only 10 to 15 IU a day. I personally take 400 IU every day. When scrutinizing this vitamin's potency, pay attention to D-alpha-tocopheryl. This is natural vitamin E. Many of the products that are sold on the market are listed as DL-alpha-tocopheryl, and that is synthetic. Try to avoid synthetic and take the natural form of E.

Fourth Commandment: Thou shall take antioxidants, especially the mineral selenium. Although heart disease is the number one killer, cancer is the one on the rise and is expected to take the first spot one of these days. A study conducted by a doctor named Larry Clark, an epidemiologist from the University of Arizona, found that when individuals with skin cancer supplemented their daily diet with 200 mcg of the essential mineral selenium, their overall risk of cancer was reduced by as much as 40-50%. Selenium is also known to reduce the risk of prostate cancer by as much as 70%, colon cancer by 60%, and lung cancer by 40%. Take heed, folks, because all these things are important for your health.

Fifth Commandment: If you are going to take only one nutrient, thou shall take vitamin E. Supplemental vitamin E is necessary since it is practically impossible to ingest the recommended amount of 100 IU from just a diet. Two studies of more than 127,000 healthcare workers, published by the *New England Journal of Medicine* and often referred to in Harvard studies, found that men and women who supplement their diets with 100 IU of vitamin E for at least two years reduce their risk of a heart attack by as much as 40%.

Sixth Commandment: Fat-soluble vitamins are nutriceuticals and thou shall consume them with low-fat meals. Since multivitamins and some nutriceuticals usually contain fat-soluble vitamins such as A, D, E, and beta-carotene (a precursor of vitamin A), it is important to take these vitamins with meals, especially with fat. If you are one of those people who skips breakfast regularly, even though you know it should be the best meal of your day, include your multivitamin or other fat-soluble dietary supplements with your lunch or dinner. If you eat a small breakfast, put a little cream cheese on a bagel or use low-fat milk with your cereal that contains nutrients that helps supplements dissolve.

Seventh Commandment: Thou shall read labels and balance the total dietary intake. If you consistently eat a healthy diet, you won't need to get 100% or more of the RDA from supplements. Too much of any good thing can be harmful and this certainly pertains to vitamins and minerals. In high doses, some can be toxic or create unpleasant side effects. It's best to keep track of your supplement quantities and make sure that they are balanced. For example, calcium and magnesium, as well as zinc and copper, should be taken together because of their biological interactions. Often when one is increased, the other is depleted. So once again, researching and keeping track of your supplements is time consuming, but it does work. Also, remember that if you are on medication of any kind, over time it will consume and destroy many of the vitamins in your body. It is important to take supplements. Talk to your doctor, and if he doesn't know which supplements to take, find someone who does.

Eighth Commandment: Remember that not all dietary supplements are created equal. As with cars and golf clubs, you usually get what you pay for. I'm not sure if that is really the way you should look at vitamins, but I have purchased many different kinds of vitamins from health food stores. Supplements from these stores are normally more expensive than grocery store vitamins and supplements that are sold in larger quantities. I believe you can get a good supplement with a good company that has a background of good products and has been around for a while. You can look on the Internet and find out just how capable these people are at producing a good product. In all cases, whenever you decide to use a certain product, look at the label carefully and ask questions if you do not understand what dosage you should take.

For instance, you may pick up two bottles of bilberry. One bottle is bilberry powder, while the other is bilberry extract. Although they may sound similar, the extract is a hundred times more potent. Both are antioxidants, which help protect the eyes against cataracts and macular degeneration caused by free radicals. So, by buying the extract you are getting a hundred times the amount of antioxidants found in the powder.

Ninth Commandment: Thou shall give dietary supplements time to work. This is a good point that I wish all of you would abide by. There are no miracles. You probably won't feel any different immediately after taking dietary supplements since it takes weeks, sometimes months, for some of the benefits to take effect. An improved immune system or increased energy levels will come with time. The important thing is to take these supplements consistently. In the case of some nutriceuticals, however, you may notice the benefits in a few days. This does not occur often, but there is that possibility.

Tenth Commandment: Thou shall design a supplement program to fit thy specific needs. Many people don't develop a program; they just throw the pills in their mouth and swallow them with a glass of water. The first step is to start on a balanced multivitamin and mineral supplement routine. The second step is to evaluate your supplement needs by looking at your family history and current health conditions, such as cholesterol and blood pressure levels. Use this list as a starting point to discuss your individual needs and dosage amounts with your healthcare provider.

For example, vitamins C, D, and E, beta-carotene, selenium, DHEA, and melatonin are all anti-aging supplements. For arthritics, the vitamin B complexes are excellent. I would take the vitamin B complex 100. Arthritic people find they can get a certain amount of relief from vitamin B complex, glucosamine sulfate, and also MSM, or methylsulfonylmethane. It takes time, but MSM is an excellent product for arthritic pain. I suggest you take it separately from glucosamine and chondroitin. I feel you can get better results from these nutrients if you take them individually.

Cancer antioxidants include selenium, bilberry extract, zinc, the B and C vitamins, and magnesium. Taking at least 750 mgs of magnesium during the course of the day does an excellent job for your eyes. It helps with heart palpitations and arrhythmia. For heart disease, one could take niacin, B6, vitamins C and E, folic acid, magnesium, L-carnitine, coenzyme Q10, hawthorne extract, copper, cortisones, and carotenes. For proper mental function, take B complexes, zinc, Ginkgo biloba (at least 120 mgs a day), phosphatidylserine, and niacinate. Acetylcholine (which is incidentally lecithin) is another wonderful product for your memory. For recall, lecithin and Ginkgo are excellent.

If you're suffering from prostate problems, take the B complexes, vitamins D and E, zinc, pumpkin seeds, pumpkin seed powder, and glycine. Pumpkin seeds are an interesting little story. People in parts of Russia and the Baltic areas have always had pumpkin seeds as a snack and eat little handfuls during the course of the day. Subsequently, in that part of the world, prostrate cancer is very rare, and this is a result of the pumpkin seeds and all the nutritional supplements they provide. I keep them as a snack on my kitchen countertop. Whenever I pass by, I eat a handful. My prostrate-specific antigen (PSA) level is just 0.1, and as you know I am eighty-one and still enjoying sex. If you have high blood pressure, I would be careful with stress, calcium, magnesium, and ginseng. Combined with a healthy diet, supplements will help your immune system and energy levels. Work out a personal plan with your physician and always seek out the latest nutritional information.

These Ten Commandments are yours to observe and apply to your good health that is within your grasp. This section is dedicated to doctors and practitioners, but mostly to medical doctors. The subject matter in this particular section is going to be dedicated to an experience I am personally involved with.

ACIDOPHILUS

This supplement is one of the many substances called probiotics, an essential form of good bacteria that provides healthy flora in the intestinal tract. The name acidophilus comes from how it produces billions of lactobacilli to fight off bad viruses and bacteria. Some practitioners believe, as well as I, that most diseases begin in the intestinal tract. Acidophilus seems to work in areas where diarrhea has discarded much of the good flora in the stomach and soothes the frequency and development of stool.

A doctor prescribes antibiotics hoping to stop a virus, and this has certainly been helpful for many. However, after working in a pharmacy for eleven years, I've noticed that doctors rarely prescribe any form of good probiotics to put back into the patient's body. They will occasionally mention such products as pure yogurt with lactobacillus or enzymes. That is my suggestion after a bout with a virus or stomach upset, even after surgery, when so many antibiotics are prescribed. Talk to a practitioner for proper dosage.

I personally take probiotics every day, just to keep my stomach relaxed and healthy. Don't forget the enzymes.

ALOE VERA

The "Hand of God" is a household plant that saves lives. This miracle product is called Aloe vera. It was used by the Egyptians and was believed to have magical healing powers. It even was assigned royal status, second only to the Pharaoh. Arab traders introduced the use of Aloe to other parts of the world. Jesuit missionaries planted it around settlements in the New World, most likely starting in Barbados in the year 1590. I cannot say enough about this beautiful supplement. It is so appealing and aesthetic to the human being, both externally and internally. Legend has it that the Indians, both in Central America and Mexico, were amazed by this plant's ability to relieve so many ailments, such as cough, abscess, arthritic pains, bursitis, cataracts, burning urine, diabetes, genital herpes, gang green, cramps, stomach pain, intestinal problems, leg ulcers, varicose veins, and yeast infections, just to name a few.

With its long leaves reaching up into Heaven, it is often called the Hand of God. An astonishing fact about this vital plant is that its reputation as a skin healer has been noted throughout the world for centuries and centuries, but what is not commonly known is that Aloe vera can be ingested in juice and capsule form. Users claim its all-natural elements regenerate internal tissue and organs the same way it regenerates the skin tissue. I can personally attest to this. I have had a stomach problem for most of my life. I even went to medical doctors with their conventional ways of treating it. Twice I had a light scope dropped down my throat and into my stomach, and nothing was ever found. After years of complaining, seeing many doctors, and taking all sorts of prescribed medicine, I finally had a decisive moment in my life when I said I just couldn't handle it anymore. I started doing some research.

To make a long story short, anyone who has a problem with their intestinal tract can now find relief. All of these things can be helped, even healed, with Aloe vera gel. That is exactly how I healed my stomach. Instead of taking all those medications, I would suggest to anyone with internal problems to try Aloe vera gel. Testimonials on the medical benefits of using Aloe vera juice internally come mostly from arthritis sufferers who claim that they now have greater mobility and relief from pain and swelling as a result of this wonder product. Others report remarkable relief from stomach ulcers and gastrointestinal problems. Some diabetics claim their need for insulin was reduced or eliminated.

Dr. Julian Whitaker is a great advocate of this particular cure. He tells the story of a ten-year-old boy who was diagnosed with a rare brain tumor. Surgeons were unable to remove the entire tumor and it continued to grow, exerting so much pressure that his eyes bulged out. The prognosis was dismal. A friend suggested that the boy drink Aloe vera concentrate. Out of desperation, the parents gave him eight ounces daily to drink. Ninety days later, to the surprise of the doctors and the elation of his family, Steve's tumor was in total remission. Today he is quite normal and continues to drink Aloe vera juice daily.

There have been innumerable miracles performed with this

particular product, and some claim that it heals cerebral palsy. Some talk about the irreversible effects of leg swelling, such as leg ulcers. An 85-year-old farmer writes that his hands pained him so much he couldn't grip anything. After a very active life, he needed help just putting on his shirt. His leg would swell up at the end of the day. He would have to get up two or three times every night to urinate, and a horrible pain struck him between his left knee and hip, forcing him to use crutches. It hurt so much that he had to lie down. However, he had to sleep sitting up because he had so much inflammation.

Then he started taking *Aloe vera* capsules, and within a week he could see a difference. He gradually got the use of his hands back. The frequent need to urinate at night stopped. His leg suddenly quit hurting. He felt good and went out and did some work on the farm. He is now able to work twelve to fourteen hours a day and says he feels like a new man. The cases go on and on. Thus, I can strongly suggest that whatever your complaint may be, you might want to try something as simplistic as taking Aloe vera juice or gel.

Elaborating a little bit further, aloe is good for people plagued with some of the following problems: hair growth, acne, sore gums, and shingles. Leg ulcers have been known to be healed, as well as bed sores and inflammatory problems if it is rubbed into the skin. It can help heal sores and burns. Please try it for healing allergies, dermatitis, and kidney infections. This powerful, viable healing plant also fights AIDS. People with AIDS say they get more relief from taking Aloe vera than they do when taking AZT, a medication.

You can grow your own aloe plant at home, and then you can bust off a piece whenever you're in need and put it on any kind of external burn or problem. As for taking it internally, I suggest you take Aloe vera gel or juice before meals and before retiring at night. As far as quantities are concerned, I think most people have to figure out which dose fits the best. I usually start off with three or four ounces twice a day. If it's for ulcers or some kind of stomach problem, I suggest taking five ounces twice a day. Do that for a couple of weeks and then gradually go down to an ounce or two a day.

AMINO ACIDS

L-carnitine is an essential amino acid. It helps with cholesterol, chronic fatigue, heart health, and lowering high blood pressure. L-carnitine is famous for aiding with chronic fatigue. How many Americans would feel better if they weren't so tired? Chronic fatigue syndrome has disabled me in many ways. I feel as though I could have been so much more successful if I had more energy. So many factors can contribute to this problem. Any time you have a weakened immune system, there is fatigue. Any time your body has to fight free radicals, heavy metal, viruses, or bacteria, you are going to sustain damage to the cells' energy factors.

There is a lot that can be done with natural substances to restore vim and vigor to every moment of our waking life. Add more fresh juices to your daily diet. Fruit juices are very beneficial, but also include lemon, lime, watermelon, and grape juice (not white grape). The juice from darker grapes seemingly has more isoflavonoids. Include soy and Aloe vera in your food selections.

Helpful herbs include garlic, St. John's wort, turmeric, echinacea, bee pollen, and Astragalus. People know when they are plagued by chronic fatigue. In fact, doctors will tell you that the principal complaint from most of their patients is that they are feeling unusually fatigued. Red clover and milk thistle are good substitutes.

For chronic fatigue, the following supplements have been found to help people: quercetin, coenzyme Q10, L-carnitine, digestive enzymes, vitamin E, and the B complex. I will always suggest that when you buy multivitamins, get the complex 100 since it covers all of the B's in 100 mgs. Vitamin C continues to be an essential!

So in your selections of supplements, look into these nutrients and follow some of these suggestions to find out which one works properly for you. I found that some of these ingredients have helped immensely with fatigue. Another amino acid that seemingly has some very promising effects is a product called L-lysine. It is an amino acid that helps women who have menopausal problems. It can rebalance hormones, thereby reducing hot flashes. Other useful supplements include dong quai, licorice root, Siberian ginseng, ginger, and a product called Schizandra. Menopausal symptoms can also be assuaged by taking vitamin C (5 to 10 grams a day), flax, and borage oil.

You want to drink a lot of berry juices. All berries, including raspberries, blueberries, cranberries, and blackberries, are rich in phytochemicals and low in calories. In addition, watermelon juice is wonderfully healthy and helpful. Other supplements to discuss with your practitioner include vitamin E and primrose oil. A lot of research has been done on primrose oil and menopause, and this product also has a tremendous effect on the ligaments in the arms, hands, and wrists. It's usually taken in an amount of 500 mgs, with 500 mgs of pantothenic acid and 3 mgs of boron. Also, you may consider calcium, magnesium citrate, L-arginine, selenium, DHEA (25 mgs), Aloe vera gel, and alpha-lipoic acid (500 mgs).

ANTIOXIDANTS

Antioxidants, as you are probably aware, secure our entire being and savage free radicals and carcinogens that can cause cancer and diseases. Antioxidants fight off all these bad little animals. I have been taking them for a number of years. I know it's worked because I haven't contracted any of these diseases. We are talking about an eighty-year-old man. Antioxidants are found in many places along the food chain. They are found freely in foods and can be isolated through pills. However, pills are a supplement and it is best if we can get all of our nutrients from plant foods, which contain thousands and thousands of antioxidants.

Free radicals that damage the cells and promote chronic disease are fought off by antioxidants. There are so many living people who have no antioxidants as a result of their food intake and who refuse to take any supplements, believing that they do not help. Whatever the reason, it is a proven fact from the *American Journal of Clinical Nutrition and Medicine* that foods and beverages from plant sources definitely provide many antioxidants. Some suggestions are blackberries, strawberries, walnuts, cranberries, artichokes, brewed coffee, raspberries, pecans, blueberries, cloves, grape juice, unsweetened baking chocolate, sour cherries, and red wine. These are in the top fifty most suggested foods to achieve maximum antioxidants. Some spices and herbs have the highest concentrations of what we need, and of course these are to be taken in smaller amounts.

Antioxidants are generally well-preserved in the process of cooking, and in fact, they actually increase with some types of cooking. For example, this happens when you boil things like carrots, spinach, mushrooms, asparagus, broccoli, cabbage, peppers, potatoes, and tomatoes in water for a few moments. You can microwave them, but I am not a proponent of microwaving. Other foods that are included in this list are kale, Brussels sprouts, cauliflower, and pomegranates. Pomegranates would probably be at the top of the list.

Many of the antioxidants that we have spoken about are present in multivitamins. They were in a mineral pill form and were developed for some people who took B vitamins, particularly thiamin, riboflavin, niacin, and B6. There are trace minerals, which also include chromium, copper, and zinc.

Here is a little tidbit for those who want to keep their complexion looking young. After I eat a piece of fruit, I rub its juices into my hands and rub it into my face in areas that I think need it. Normally people would go to the sink and wash the juice off with cold or warm water and soap. The acids in fruits and vegetables have a tremendous effect upon skin. When in need, use the meat of fruit. The skin on the inside of the banana does wonders for your face. When you're eating an apple and you get it on the side of your face and wipe it off, wipe it into your skin. Any kind of juice has a tremendous amount of acidity which influences the collagen in your skin. Just thought you might like to know!

ASTRAGALUS

Astragalus is a Chinese tonic. Asians have been consuming this herb for more than 5,000 years. Chinese practitioners prescribe this herb for many ailments and believe its contents are better than all others in fighting most diseases. This includes cancer, arthritis, bone growth, diabetes, lung disease, and heart disease, just to mention a few. Astragalus gets the most attention for its super ability to support the immune system. Asians believe it has thousands of years to show for it, because when our immune system is high, we can fight all diseases much more effectively.

It has been my experience that Astragalus is not a quick fix. To achieve maximum healing results, the herb must be taken in quantities of 400 to 800 mgs up to three times a day. After thirty days, patients seem to have more energy and the feeling of better health. There have been no ill side effects if taken six months or more. Postoperative people seem to recover in less time opposed to those who have not taken the herb. Talk to your practitioner for the correct dosage.

CALCIUM

Calcium is an essential vitamin for your bone structure. It helps to prevent osteoporosis and arteriosclerosis. Also, calcium often is not very absorbable; therefore, there are vitamin supplements that contain a form of vitamin D, which is a form of pure sunshine. Vitamin D is an essential vitamin that needs to go into your body with calcium to make it absorbable. There are different ways of taking calcium. I take it all the time; however, with the size of some of these tablets that are on the market today, there are many people who just won't take them. I have suggested that these people take the supplement by putting the tablets in some water and letting them dissolve a little, and then swallowing them. But for the most part, people want to do it the easy way.

Calcium is something that many women do not take. I know of many women who are hunched over and can hardly walk and whose joints are swollen because of rheumatoid arthritis. I've been to a couple of classes on rheumatoid arthritis. It's a terrible disease which will eventually kill you if it gets bad enough. There are some modern medicines out there, so if the calcium doesn't work, people who are in a lot of pain will end up taking anything. There are a couple of drugs out there that will fry your brain and make you even worse. I am not mentioning any names because someone would sue me for sure. Working in the pharmacy made me aware that this medication just causes an enormous amount of problems, and even in the class that I took, they showed how harmful it is and what it does over a period of time. It destroys your innards.

The best approach is to first increase your calcium by eating the right kinds of food. This includes low-fat milk and low-fat organic proteins that are on the market today. There are many excellent products on the market that consist of purified organic soy. I take it every day on my cereal. I personally do not drink milk anymore, especially if it is homogenized. There are just too many ways of collecting bacteria, and I don't want to deal with that. Taking calcium is a very important factor like everything else.

When reading this, a lot of people are probably going to say, "I don't have time to take all the supplements," or "I don't want to." That is entirely up to you. My only suggestion is that when you have a problem, you want to try to correct it before it gets worse. When considering my suggestions, remember that I have personally taken these products. I know that they work, not only because they help me, but because they also help my patients.

You need to know what to get and how to buy it, and then need to make sure that you take it. If you don't take it, it isn't going to work. The same thing happens when you go to the medical doctor. He gives you a prescription, you take it, and it knocks you on your fanny. You know it doesn't work, or if it does work, you now have exchanged one symptom for another. That is what prescription medications do—treat the symptoms. The things that I am suggesting here go back thousands and thousands of years. They work, and I can vouch for it. I have never had surgery. I have been to the doctor a number of times because I did not know what to do many years ago. When they weren't helping me, I decided to go a different route and try to inform others.

Calcium can be acquired through many forms of good food. A lot of the nutrients in food have fatty substances but are very good for you. For example, nuts have a lot of calcium, such as peanuts, cashews, and walnuts. They are a good source of omega-3 fatty acids. They do have some fat content, but if you exercise regularly, that should not be a factor. I exercise daily, some days more than others, but I do not have any fat on my body that I am aware of. Sometimes if I feel like I am getting a little bit heavier, I just don't eat as much or I cut down on some of the things I think might be fattening. It's just that simple.

COENZYME Q10

This product has helped me immensely. I mentioned earlier in the book that I have had a heart palpitation for a long time. I went to many doctors, and most of them wanted to load me up with all kinds of medications. I tried a few and they literally gave me no energy and just knocked me out. Worse yet, they didn't really help with the heart palpitations. Sometimes my heart would feel as though it skipped and it would leave me breathless at times. This would make me feel panicky, and when I got breathless, it would make me very upset.

I had been taking potassium, magnesium, and calcium, and it did help a lot. That's when I did some research on coenzyme Q10, which has been out for a number of years now. I started taking coenzyme Q10 about three and a half years ago. I have found that it not only helps to regulate my heart but also infiltrates my entire body with Q10. It helps me to think better, and it helps my blood flow. Coenzyme Q10 is just a magnificent supplement. *Life Extension* magazine has put out a tremendous article on it, including how it contributes to a man's heart muscle. It actually helps to repair it. Coenzyme Q10 is present in every cell in our body, including the mitochondria. It circulates throughout your entire system and regulates your body. It has regulated my heart, and when I don't take it, I can certainly feel the difference.

I would recommend coenzyme Q10 for people who have allergies, Alzheimer's, or for the prevention of Alzheimer's. I also recommend it for arthritis, chronic fatigue syndrome, digestive disorders, emphysema, energizing brain cells, free radical activity, and heart health. There also is a strong possibility that it helps lower high blood pressure. For Parkinson's disease, it has been noted to help many people. It is an excellent product and I recommend it highly for anybody with the above problems. The dosage is going to have to be experimental between you and your practitioner. The dosage that I personally take is as follows: I started off at 300 mgs a day and have ultimately come down to about 100 mgs per day. I find this dose to be substantial enough for my benefit and helpful in what I am trying to accomplish. I use it for my heart issues, and I have that particular problem squared away with the magnesium, potassium, and calcium. But the thing that put the cap on it was the coenzyme Q10.

Most of your good cardiologists today will recommend it for people with heart problems, since it can give you a stronger heart and a healthier life. Again, for the best results, contact your practitioner or someone knowledgeable who can give you some information about the best dosage for you. Unfortunately, coenzyme Q10 is not inexpensive. I have found that the best source of coenzyme Q10 runs anywhere from $22 to $26 for 100 mgs, which is thirty gels. Incidentally, I would strongly suggest taking the gel capsules—the orange-colored ones are the best. There is a powder form, but it is not as effective as the gel form. Gel capsules are the best approach, but again, they're on the expensive side and I haven't seen them come down in price in the last three years. In fact, if anything, the price has gone up.

If you have a problem with your heart, I strongly suggest that you give coenzyme Q10 a shot. It worked for me and hopefully it will work for you.

ECHINACEA

Echinacea is essential to the immune system. It boosts the immune system activity and promotes fast recovery, especially when taken at the onset of symptoms, such as a cold or flu virus. Most potent formulas have a peculiar tingling and numbing effect on the tongue since the body cannot sustain such high levels of echinacea in the immune system. Echinacea should not be used for any long period of time. It should be taken in short intervals when the symptoms occur. In most cases, echinacea should only be taken on a six-week basis and then stopped to let the immunity build up.

In Europe, for example, they have a system where echinacea is used extensively and people take the herb in a pattern that consists of four days on and four days off, which gives it time to regenerate itself. It seems that echinacea yields no more benefits after it has been used continuously for six weeks. You need to stop for at least a month and then you can go back to it. Dosage intervals depend upon the individual, but when you buy echinacea at the health food store, you should pay attention to the suggested amounts. If this is not enough, it is not harmful to take more. Hopefully echinacea can successfully enhance your immune system when you need it.

FOLIC ACID

Folic acid helps maintain normal levels of serotonin. Deficiencies contribute to depression, dementia, and schizophrenia. Taking folic acid helps prevent heart attacks. How beautiful it would be if people suffering from depression and other mental problems could be advised to try the B complex before taking antidepressants, which are loaded with side effects. My suggestion to most of my patients is to take a 100 mg complex, and include 800 mcg of folic acid with 1,000 mcg of B12 daily. B12 is recommended, and I take it each morning before I run. I have an easier run and feel less fatigue. It's an inexpensive way of improving your health and getting more energy in your life. A combination of 1,000 mcg B12 and 800 mcg folic acid before a run can make your workout more enjoyable. You should enjoy everything you do; otherwise, it will likely be less effective.

Much has been written about how folic acid helps prevent birth defects, especially spina bifida. I have witnessed the tragedy of spina bifida and it's not pretty. If pregnant, talk to your practitioner regarding the quantity you should consume.

GINKGO BILOBA

I would like to elaborate on what I have previously mentioned regarding Ginkgo. Over the last eighty-five years, the E Commission in Germany has researched and made many improvements in what we can do to expedite our good health. This includes taking Ginkgo. It has been in existence since the beginning of time and even survived the ice age.

Ginkgo has lasting effects on the body. It improves circulation in all the vital tissues and organs, such as the heart and the brain. It helps to protect our organs from potentially dangerous chemicals called free radicals. It blocks a substance in our bodies called the platelet-activating factor (PAF), which may contribute to asthma, heart disease, hearing disorders, and skin disorders such as psoriasis. Ginkgo may be an ideal herbal support to counteract some of the most common conditions associated with the aging process and with environmental pollution and stress. With regular use, Ginkgo can help increase and maintain blood supply to all the tissues of the body, but most especially to the brain, extremities, skin, eyes, inner ears, heart, and other vital organs. Major uses of Ginkgo are for brain function. Decreased blood flow to the brain can adversely affect memory, concentration, intellectual ability, vision, equilibrium, and balance, and may also lead to symptoms such as headache, depression, and mental confusion. Ginkgo is used to prevent and even treat all of these conditions.

Circulation disorders, such as peripheral vascular disease, may lead to poor circulation in the legs, making it difficult to walk. They also cause poor circulation to the skin, heart, and other organs. Regarding hearing disorders, at the pharmacy, many people would complain that their doctor-prescribed drugs were not working. I suggested that they start taking 120 to 220 mgs of Ginkgo per day. Without exception, every single one of them had a depletion or complete annihilation of their tinnitus (ringing in the ears).

Disturbance of balance, dizziness, vertigo, sudden hearing loss, and hearing weaknesses may result from a lack of proper blood circulation. Ginkgo has been a great support to these types of diseases. These conditions may also be caused by free radical damage.

Eye disorders are another area where Ginkgo does a fabulous job. The retina may be damaged by free radicals. Hemorrhaging can occur, and stress factors in our everyday lives can restrict circulation. Alzheimer's is one of the diseases that all of us fear as we age. We wonder why we forget some things so easily. Ginkgo protects against brain weaknesses. It improves the blood circulation and protects against free radical damage.

Ginkgo improves the condition of the blood. It thins the blood viscosity and lowers platelet adhesiveness, protects red blood cells from stabilizing their membranes, increases blood flow and vessel tone, stabilizes capacity, and also stabilizes capillary unity.

Ginkgo protects brain cell membranes and other tissues throughout the body against any free radical damage. Cell membranes are particularly sensitive to free radical damage, and this can lead to the destruction of the entire cell. Ginkgo increases the uptake and utilization of oxygen and glucose in tissues throughout the body. It increases the blood flow to the brain and extremities, and it regulates our increased brain metabolism. This counteracts depression without a doubt. I know that Ginkgo has helped me in the past with depression, and I continue taking it each and every day. It regulates the neurotransmitters that guard against memory loss, depression, and senility. It protects myelin that coats the nerves against some kinds of damage. It helps protect hearing, and even restores impaired hearing, especially due to damage from loud noise or infection. Also, it slows certain bacterial activity. Based on my own experiences, I greatly recommend this supplement. You can take as much as 320 mgs of Ginkgo without having any side effects. I have personally taken that much when my health was poor. Each and every one of us has changes in our chemical production over a period of time. Consider Ginkgo as your primary interest each and every day.

Start out small, around 120 mgs, and you can work up from there if needed.

Ginkgo does a large amount of good for you and me. It is a significant ingredient in the multivitamin I have on the market. Around the world, Ginkgo is taken to boost circulation and help force off mental decline. Ginkgo, which is also an antioxidant, is used in China and Germany to alleviate dizziness and memory problems. A study by the New York Institute of Medical Research on people in the beginning stages of Alzheimer's found that Ginkgo could slightly slow the progress of this devastating disease. To further the study of possible benefits of Ginkgo, the Office of Alternative Medicine and the National Institute on Aging are currently finishing up a study in Oregon's Health University in Portland. This is being done with about three dozen people with early Alzheimer's, and the results of the research should be available in the next few years.

LECITHIN

Lecithin is a powerful nutritional product. It comes from soy, which I am sure you have heard so many wonderful things about. Like anything else, it needs to be taken in moderation. You should realize that you can overdo anything. I don't care if you're eating spinach, you can overdo it. Too much of anything is not good.

Lecithin is a powerful stimulus for your mind and body. I have been taking it for a long period of time and can personally say it has an immediate positive effect on my remembering abilities. Lecithin is a natural food. Your doctor would probably suggest it if he were discussing beneficial substances for the brain, nervous system, cardiovascular system, liver, and other vital parts of your body. There is no other nutrient that is more prominent in this area.

Lecithin is found in every living cell. Its highest concentration is in the vital living organs: the brain, the heart, the liver, and the kidneys. Our brains have a dry composition of 30% lecithin. It performs an astonishing range of essential functions directly affecting our health and wellbeing. In the brain, lecithin choline is transformed into what is known as acetylcholine. This is a vital compound for the transmission of messages from one nerve to another. It has a proven effect on memory, thinking ability, and muscle control. In the blood stream, lecithin helps to prevent cholesterol and other unwanted fats from accumulating on the artery walls. It may help dissolve deposits from arteries that are somewhat clogged up already. In the liver, lecithin metabolizes clogged fat and reduces the chance of liver degeneration. In the intestinal tract, the absorption of the vitamins A and D influences the utilization of other fat-soluble nutrients such as vitamins E and K. The list goes on and on. I am mostly interested in lecithin because of the brainpower it seems to magnify. There is no question about it—lecithin definitely gives you a better mind, and when your mind is good, you will definitely have a longer lifespan.

This brain tonic has an interesting background. In 1975, scientists at the Massachusetts Institute of Technology discovered that lecithin choline has a prompt effect on the brain's ability to make an important chemical called acetylcholine. The most surprising part of the discovery was that choline is taken up by the brain directly from the circulatory blood. It has long been believed that something called the blood-brain barrier protects the brain from such direct influences. Only a few substances, notably alcohol and narcotics, are heretofore known to be able to penetrate the barrier. This means that each time you take lecithin it has an immediate effect on the production of chemicals that are essential for signal transmission in the brain.

Regarding dosage, you should take the amount of lecithin described on the product label. Try to get the good form of lecithin at your health food store. Just because it costs more doesn't necessarily mean it's better for you. Check it out, and do a little research. You can buy lecithin in grain form and put it in your cereal, or you can buy it in capsule form. The normal dosage is around 1,000 to 2,000 mgs. Soy lecithin normally is around 1,200 to 1,500 mgs per day. Give it a try; it will definitely help you to think better, especially if you are a student. Lecithin and Ginkgo are two of the most mind-exhilarating nutrients you can put into your body. As I said before, I have taken all of these, and when I was at school, especially during the time of exams, I would take lecithin and Ginkgo about an hour or two before the tests and they helped remarkably. Give it a shot.

There are other ingredients that you should take along with lecithin to achieve optimal supplementation, such as magnesium, potassium, zinc, and chromium. There is another product on the market called phosphate L-serine (PS), a fatty compound found in small quantities. It has recently emerged as a promising candidate for improving overall age-related mental decline. PS acts in the brain at the level of the nerve cell membrane, regulating nerve impulses. PS normally occurs fossilized in the brain tissue. Lecithin produces two chemicals called inositol and choline, which are neurotransmitters to the brain. These products help to sharpen your mind and give you the brainpower you need to exist in our environment. You will better remember new tasks. For instance, to learn new programs on the computer, you might practice them daily over a course of a few weeks. When you do this, you will find a great deal of difference in the way you think.

Don't forget to exercise to boost your circulation and keep your body and mind in a functional order. Vitamins C and E are essential, along with selenium. I take these products every single day, and they are included in a product that I have on the market. I personally don't think you can get everything you need from one pill, so you need to supplement extra amounts of vitamins C and E into your regimen. In terms of vitamin E, make sure that you take D-alpha-tocopheryl, rather that the DL form. DL is synthetic and doesn't have the same effectiveness as D-alpha-tocopheryl. All in all, I am not suggesting substituting anything for medications prescribed by your physician. Always get the okay or tell your doctor what you are taking. This is essential.

MAGNESIUM

Magnesium is probably one of the most necessary minerals to our existence. Over two million Americans experience an irregular or abnormal heartbeat called arrhythmia. Orthodox medicines offer an impressive and intimidating array of high-tech treatments for arrhythmia, including prescription drugs to regulate the heartbeat and surgery to excise heart tissue where arrhythmia originates. Diagnosing arrhythmia is contingent upon a number of factors including associated symptoms and the patient's age. As we get older, our heartbeat usually decreases. Arrhythmia is characterized by the type of erratic heartbeat and the location of where these beats originate in the heart. Physicians determine this by using an electrocardiograph.

Two of the deadliest arrhythmias are tachycardia and ventricular fibrillation. These types can be fatal if the heart rate exceeds one-hundred beats per minute. This commonly leads to ventricular fibrillation, and the heart artery blockage frequently collapses and people die. While the victim can sometimes be revived by CPR, death is likely unless the underlying electrical problems are treated immediately.

This is where magnesium comes into play for those who prefer alternative medicines. Over the past few years, a safe, natural solution for many types of arrhythmia has been gaining national attention: magnesium. Consider magnesium supplements instead of cardiac drugs. It seems ironic that the very drugs that are used to treat heart problems such as arrhythmia can also cause arrhythmia. Digitalis, for example, is a powerful drug derived from the leaves of foxglove, which works by blocking sodium potassium. Digitalis stimulates heart function and can save lives in conjunctive heart failure patients. There is a catch, however. Digitalis interferes with the normal roles that magnesium and potassium play. Without magnesium, the body cannot utilize potassium. Therefore, a magnesium deficiency equates to a potassium deficiency. By using digitalis, the heart cells become more excitable and more prone to arrhythmia. Drugs given to treat heart failure and high blood pressure, such as diuretics and thiazide, also quickly deplete magnesium and potassium. A magnesium deficiency can occur when a physician prescribes drugs such as quinidine sulfate and diisopropylamide phosphate to treat arrhythmia.

With the knowledge of magnesium benefits on the rise, more and more physicians are advocating its use in heart disease therapy. Numerous medical studies down-stating the value of magnesium, particularly in cases of arrhythmia, have made more believers than skeptics. It just so happens that I once had an arrhythmia problem which has been totally alleviated by taking magnesium, potassium, and calcium. Magnesium is vital to enzyme activity and acts like a starter to some of the chemical reactions in the body. It assists in calcium and potassium uptake and plays an important role as coenzyme in the building of protein. This essential mineral protects the arterial lining from sudden blood pressure changes and plays an important role in the formation of bone. About 70% of magnesium is located in the bones and the remaining 30% is found in the soft tissue and blood. For healthy individuals, the daily requirement for magnesium is between 200 and 500 mgs. If a diet is rich in dark green vegetables, raw nuts and seeds, grapefruit, corn, and figs, one might be getting the necessary amount of magnesium.

There are other factors that can lead to a magnesium deficiency in spite of a good diet. As we age, our systems often aren't as efficient as they once were, or the food we eat may be lacking in magnesium due to poor soil. Some common symptoms of magnesium deficiency include kidney stones, charley horses, cramps, bone spurs, nervous twitching, and, of course, arrhythmia. Magnesium's usefulness to treat arrhythmia was first reported in 1915. Since that time, scores of clinical studies supporting its benefits have been published in medical journals. However, doctors still reject the idea, not because they object to taking magnesium, but because they feel as though they are not knowledgeable enough to prescribe the adequate dosages since they don't study that aspect of it. This is unfortunate. By taking magnesium instead of drugs, you eliminate most side effects.

Remember, taking large doses of magnesium over a long period of time can probably have some toxicity, but never enough to kill you. The body uses magnesium to calm the nervous system. Normally, for someone who has an arrhythmia, probably 1,000 mgs of magnesium, about 2,000 mgs of potassium, and about 1,500 mgs of calcium a day would be beneficial. All of these should be taken at the same time because they are very synergistic and work well together. A magnesium deficiency can cause a muscular problem or nervous insomnia because one of its functions is to relax muscles and quiet nerves. Magnesium is also useful in the prevention of kidney stones. Basically, kidney stones from urinary calcium don't remain dissolved. Instead, they form small pellets made from the calcium salts.

In conclusion, since 1988, there has been a renowned interest in this mighty mineral following a symposium in New York City that focused strictly on magnesium. Its importance shouldn't be underestimated since it is safe as well as extremely beneficial to your entire being.

I would like to also give a little information on how to prevent leg cramps. A natural prescription would be to eliminate as much sugar and caffeine from your diet as possible. This is in addition to taking daily supplements. This has worked for my family and for me. Take 1,200 mgs of calcium at bedtime. Make sure you are getting 1,200 mgs of calcium daily through your diet and other supplements. For pregnant women, check with your doctor before beginning supplementation. Also, take 400 IU of vitamin E twice a day after meals for two weeks. If symptoms are relieved, cut the dosage down to 400 IU once a day. If symptoms reoccur, the dosage can be increased, but never take more than 1,200 IU daily. You can take up to 1,000 mgs of magnesium. Take it in dosages intermittently from morning until night along with your calcium. Take 10,000 IU of vitamin A daily, or take beta-carotene (a precursor for vitamin A), and 100 mgs of potassium. These work tremendously well.

SELENIUM

Selenium is an essential trace mineral for both humans and animals. It was discovered in 1817 by a Swedish chemist, Jons Jakob Berzelius, who named the trace mineral "selenium" after a moon goddess. Selenium originates in the soil, where it is absorbed by plants. Plants in turn are consumed by living organisms, and so it moves up into the food chain. Therefore, one would assume that selenium is always present in the food chain products we consume. Thus, many believe that a shortage of selenium in a human diet would be a rare occurrence.

Unfortunately for many, a deficiency of selenium happens all too often. This occurs because in many parts of the world, the soil is deficient in this mineral. It wasn't until 1957 that Dr. Klaus Schwartz determined selenium to be an essential element for animals. Its essentiality in the human diet took another sixteen years to be discovered.

It was at the University of Wisconsin where doctors demonstrated that selenium was absorbed into the molecules of an enzyme called glutathione. This enzyme is essential for the protection of red blood cells, cell membranes, and sub-cellular components against dangerous reactions with soluble pesticides.

In short, it is an effective antioxidant. This discovery led to the understanding that the new selenium protects us against cancer, heart disease, arthritis, and an accelerated amount of aging devices. In fact, evidence exists that shows selenium may even cure many types of cancer. While it is true that selenium by itself cannot prevent or protect all people from all types of cancer, it definitely reduces the risk of cancer.

Selenium also plays an important role in the muscle function of the heart. It was first studied in animals. Human studies have been conducted that test the protective and therapeutic roles selenium plays on the heart. It is interesting to note why many people are deficient in this particular mineral. One of the reasons people pray for floods from rivers and the like is because it appears to wash all of the nutrients back into the soil. When there are no floods, such as in the middle part of the United States, the water does not accumulate for many years. Since there are no minerals and nutrients being washed into the area, the soil where different vegetables and fruits are grown produces no selenium. When there are no flooding waters, there is no selenium.

In certain countries, such as Asia, selenium is present in high levels because continuous floods hit the area. For example, this happens around the Nile River, which floods maybe two or three times a year. There is heavy selenium production in that area. It just goes to show that even though people sometimes don't like floods, there is a purpose behind why God puts them there.

There are many types of selenium, and the organic form is preferred due to its bioavailability to the body. You need to get the most organic bioavailable type of selenium. It is a similar to the essential amino acid methionine but has an atom of selenium instead of an atom of sulfur. It better absorbs and is better incorporated into the body components than any other form of selenium. In fact, experiments have revealed that this form of organic selenium is actually five times more bioavailable than the inorganic form. Worldwide research is revealing that selenium is more than just an important nutrient; it is an insurance policy on which daily premiums should be paid. Some women's diseases can also be prevented. The most prevalent is the one that everyone seems to be discussing more so than ever: breast cancer. Selenium, as I said, plays a vital role in the prevention of heart disease and many forms of cancer, and this possibly includes breast cancer.

Proper use of selenium can also slow the aging process, strengthen the immune system, and improve energy levels. There is increasing evidence that selenium can help prevent and relieve arthritis, forestall the onset of cataracts, and improve resistance to infectious diseases. One of the things that is so beautiful about selenium is that it protects the membranes that are in each of our bodies—that's sixty trillion cells. Dr. Passwater of the University of Philadelphia says that it prevents the decay of your cellular functions. The average reader will appreciate the role selenium plays in protecting the body against a whole host of diseases. Selenium's effectiveness has been repeatedly demonstrated in different laboratories around the world. Know that selenium is protective against cancer, heart disease, and premature aging.

Selenium is a giant step toward preventing cancer. Recently, several physicians have found that when sufficient selenium is ingested by cancer patients wishing to raise their blood levels of selenium to a desired range, their tumors began to shrink. The University of California claims that if every woman in America started taking selenium today, or had a high selenium diet, the breast cancer rate in this country would drastically decline within a few years. If selenium were used properly as a protective measure against cancer, it is possible that it would enable us to cut the mortality rate from almost all cancers by as much as 80-90% in this country.

Based on epidemiological studies, one of the doctors in the Cleveland Clinic Foundation advises people to increase their intake of selenium to 200 mcg a day. It can reduce the cancer rate dramatically for some types of cancer, particularly cancer of the colon, breast, esophagus, tongue, stomach, intestines, rectum, and bladder. Selenium is necessary for the health of the heart muscle itself. Selenium supplementation is effective in the treatment of chest pain associated with the heart disease angina pectoris.

Chinese physicians recently reported that cognitive heart disease, one that affects children especially, was prominent throughout vast regions of China. Since this land is known to be low in selenium, physicians set up a carefully controlled study and found that when people were given 1,000 mcg of selenium each week, before long the incidents of the heart problem, called Keshan disease, dropped to zero. The children who were already suffering from heart trouble became well. This is amazing news.

Those who become educated about taking selenium daily are going to be healthier and stronger, have a better immune system, and also live longer. Selenium and vitamin E are required to produce the coenzyme Q10 in the body. Dr. Passwater tells the story of Mrs. X. She went to the clinic and a biopsy showed she had a late stage of incurable muscular dystrophy. She was told to go home because nothing could be done. A friend of hers, however, was a medical researcher who felt that the muscular dystrophy was due to the lack of coenzyme Q10. She increased vitamin B, even taking 400 to 2,000 IU, and vitamin C, taking 3,000 mgs a day. She went on a diet rich in cottage cheese and tuna fish to supply selenium. Her triglycerides dropped from 130 to 68, her cholesterol dropped from 240 to 186, and her creatine phosphokinase (CPK), an important indicator of MD, dropped from 610 to 140, which is considered borderline with respect to MD. Dr. Passwater says that nutritional MD in animals is different than the MD in humans, but maybe not if some patients respond to selenium plus vitamin E or coenzyme Q10 therapy.

Dr. Gerald Schwarhouser is quoted in one of Dr. Richard Passwater's books as saying that the preferred dietary sources of selenium are whole wheat breads, cereals, and organ meats like liver, kidneys, and seafood. Well, I don't think there's going to be too many people rushing out to eat liver and kidneys, so supplementations should take care of that. A pill containing 150 to 200 mcg of selenium will provide good maintenance for all ages.

Dr. Schwarhouser says he personally takes 200 mcg of selenium per day. Occasionally, he increases this to 300 or 400. There will be no toxicity problems with a regular dose of 800 mcg per day, even over extended periods. You can take 2,000 mcg for some time without harm, but this is about the limit. All in all, selenium is a very safe supplement capable of preventing the above diseases and giving you a better life.

TAURINE

Taurine is an amino acid. It is one of the many supplements I ingest for an improved mind. It has a sulfur compound that assists in the treatment of a number of disorders. Taurine also prevents Alzheimer's and dementia and serves as the antioxidant that protects the supply of magnesium and calcium within the brain cells. It also enhances nerve cell functioning.

This supplement can help fortify cardiac contractions and enhance the outflow of blood from the heart. A normal dose of taurine at 500 mgs two times a day may be a key factor in avoiding congestive heart failure and arterioscleroses. This amino acid is a free form that participates in a variety of metabolic processes. Taurine is a neurotransmitter and a neuromodulator and is involved in glucose uptake. It is found in meats, fish, milk, and eggs, but not in vegetable proteins, so supplementation is especially important for vegetarians. These supplements are best absorbed with food. When I'm nervous or upset, 500 mgs of taurine taken two times a day settles my mind and body. It's much safer than antidepressants, and has no side effects.

THYROXINE

Thyroxine is a substitute hormone for your thyroid gland. This amino acid is used when the gland is unable to produce as much as it should. An alternative substitute for thyroxine might be suitable. Thyroxine also is acceptable for people with high blood pressure. Alternative treatment includes detoxification, diet improvement, and stress reduction. Some holistic physicians may give patients a natural form of thyroid hormone replacement which has side effects over time. Thyroxine acts as a neurotransmitter to the brain. Many alternative practitioners suggest using it to treat depression. Thyroxine has helped me, and when I feel better, I discontinue its use. Your practitioner will help you figure out what is best for your body.

VITAMIN B

The B vitamins consist of thiamin (B1), riboflavin (B2), niacin pyridoxine (B6), folic acid, pantothenic acid, biotin, and cobalamin (B12). All play an enormously huge role on the brain waves, functioning of neurotransmitters, and regulating energy to our brain cells.

Severe vitamin B deficiencies have been shown to lead to abnormal brain waves. This can cause impaired memory and higher levels of anxiety, confusion, irritability, and depression. Even marginal deficiencies of vitamin B can cause EEG disturbances and inhibit mental performance (this has been researched at the Human Nutrition Center in North Dakota). Many of the studies involved older people who are frequently deficient in vitamins and minerals, but the same could be expected from younger people lacking in B nutrition.

Studies show thiamine deficiency hampers the brain's ability to use glucose, decreases energy available for mental activities, and overexcites neurons so they fire endlessly, poop out, and die. Even if you are marginally deficient in thiamine, you may be slowing down your brain power.

VITAMIN C

Vitamin C, or ascorbic acid, can be bought with bio-flavonoids, which are comprised of the B complexes. However, I take the nutrient separately. I do not take the combinations of vitamins that are suggested by some manufacturers. I think there is less potency when you take them in combinations, even in multivitamins. There is no way in the world you can fill a small pill with all the ingredients supposedly contained in that product. I'm not denying that it isn't there, but it is just not enough in most instances. Vitamin C is without a doubt the most prominent vitamin of all. There are five essentials that are vital to your health, and vitamin C happens to be one of them. The others are A, B, E, and selenium. Vitamin C covers a category of almost every disease that the human body is prone to.

There is another essential benefit to vitamin C that most people don't consider, and that's the skin. I take 3,000 mgs of vitamin C ascorbic acid and mix it in a container with about four or five ounces of water. I then rub it on my face with moisturizers of some form. You can even use cocoa butter. I also use vitamin C after I shave. The collagen that it puts in your skin and body is incredible. That is why it is essential that you take it both internally and externally. It will help over a period of time to eliminate brown spots on your face and hands. It can also help treat many other forms of diseases.

I'm going to give you an idea of the many other benefits of vitamin C. One of them involves bioflavonoids, which reduce cholesterol and help eliminate bleeding gums. Vitamin C is excellent for your eyes. Most research shows that it definitely prevents cataracts. It also works well for people who have headaches, heat rashes, hemorrhoids, spider bites, and sunburned eyes. It can be used as a night cream. Vitamin C helps to prevent nose bleeds. It also helps with smoking. For every cigarette you smoke, 500 mgs of vitamin C are extracted from your body.

It is essential to have vitamin C in your body, and it can be collected through many sources of fruits and vegetables. You can get much more if you take it internally as a nutrient. My suggestion is to take 3,000 mgs of vitamin C every day. If you notice you have an oncoming flu, cold, or virus of some nature, or just don't feel too well in general, you can take as much as 10,000 mgs per day. Remember that Linus Pauling, who received two Nobel Prizes, believed in the definite correlation of vitamin C and good health, and also the extraction and prevention of many diseases. I personally take about 4,000 mgs of vitamin C every single day. This is part of the reason why I have such excellent health. When I don't feel up to par, or I feel like I'm catching something, I extend my vitamin C intake. It definitely gives me energy and helps my immune system, which is the most important thing of all.

Something needs to be mentioned about vitamin C. Regardless of how much you take throughout the day, please understand that it is water soluble. Therefore, when you urinate, have a bowel excretion, or perspire, vitamin C will disappear from your body. Subsequently, you have to take it intermittently all day long. Your body will use more of it that way, and you will also prevent urinary tract irritation. Vitamin B is water soluble and does the same thing. So you need to take these things all day long in small doses.

Another thought: If you are taking vitamin C in the form of a capsule, that should be okay since it's absorbable. If you are taking a pill, I suggest you put it in a little bit of water and let it soak for a couple of hours. If you find that it is not breaking up, the pill is going to do the same thing in your body. It's not going to do anything, and it is going to pass right though. So test all of your pills and make sure you are getting the best absorption when you take them.

For best results, it would be even better to put the vitamin C in some vinegar. About an inch or half-inch in a bottle is okay. Vinegar acts like stomach acid and will help break down the vitamin in the same way. In fact, this is true of any form of medication you may be taking. Vinegar ensures that you get the right amount of absorption.

You can also determine whether or not your nutrients are being absorbed by observing your bowel movements. See if the bowel movement makes a mark on the toilet bowl. Stools that adhere to the surface of a toilet bowl and make a mark indicate faulty digestive capacity. This is usually because it is made up of fat. Thus, it doesn't matter if you have the best diet in the world; if it is not processed and absorbed properly, you are just not getting the full benefits. So take heed and notice what your stool is doing. A bowel movement alleviates all of the food and undesirable absorption in your system. This is the greatest thing in the world. Research has shown that two to three bowel movements a day is best. Be sure that your vitamin C and other nutrients are being absorbed properly.

ZINC

This is another mineral that I take every day. If you are looking for healthier skin on your entire body, you should try zinc. Remember that your skin is the largest organ of your body. Zinc is an essential trace element involved in many human biological functions, including cell division. Zinc will reciprocate the process of aging well. An antioxidant, zinc protects against macular degeneration—an age-related vision impairment. Arthritis responds to zinc supplements. In one study, 220 mgs of zinc was given three times a day for twelve weeks to rheumatoid arthritis patients. They reported feeling significant improvement in their joints and walking time, and the swelling and morning stiffness decreased.

Cancer is another area where zinc is considered an important element, as long as it's taken in trace amounts. Cancer patients taking 250 mgs of oral zinc gluconate for three weeks showed enhanced immune function. Animal studies suggest that zinc may prevent heart disease and stroke and mitigate the negative effects of chronic stress. Also, zinc shows promise in male infertility.

Studies point to zinc in the treatment of skin disorders, such as eczema, herpes, and acne. I recently had a skin inflammation on my face. During this time, I increased my zinc intake, and over a period of about ten days, it subsided and healed. Many people have anorexic symptoms because they do not have zinc in their normal diet. Zinc doses begin at 49 mgs a day. It helps anorexic patients to gain weight. Zinc also aids patients with sickle cell anemia, cerebral palsy, and inflammatory bowel disease.

SECTION 4
AGING

OVERVIEW

There are many myths about aging that I think I should discuss briefly. Americans seem to be bent on denying the aging process. Ours is a youthful society, with images of pubescent youngsters dominating the media. Even as awareness on aging increases, most magazines, films, and television programs portray vital older people. Culturally, we also carry around negative stereotypes of aging people. No wonder we fear our own aging. I've often said, "If I didn't know how old I was, I wouldn't know how old I was." Growing older cannot be avoided, but it doesn't have to mean a loss of physical or mental health.

In fact, research indicates that just the opposite is true. By paying attention to lifestyle as we age, most of us can live an active and healthy life that shatters the old-age myths. Ask your doctor about nutrition supplements and dietary changes. I hope you go to a doctor who entertains the idea of herbs, vitamins, and supplements in your life. If he doesn't, I would switch doctors. An old proverb says, "The older I get, the sicker I get." However, old age isn't tantamount to illness.

An important part of staying well in your older years is keeping your immune system healthy. One way to achieve this is to take nutritional supplements. When healthy elderly people were fed nutritional supplements for a year, their immune systems improved, according to a Johns Hopkins University study. Those who took supplements in the place of a placebo were plagued with fewer infections and had to take antibiotics for fewer days. You should note that these effects were achieved with regular amounts of nutrients in a balanced formula. Mega-doses are not always good for you. In addition to keeping the immune system operating at peak performance, changes targeted at specific diseases can help us with illness as we age. Evidence shows that high potassium, salt restriction, weight maintenance, and dietary supplements of calcium and magnesium can help control hypertension.

Smoking and low plasma levels of vitamin C, vitamin E, and beta-carotene contribute to cataracts. According to the *Journal of American Medical Association*, quitting smoking and eating a diet rich in nutrients helps to reduce the risk of these conditions. Adult-onset diabetes and cancer may be prevented by changes in diet. Records estimate that half of all illnesses are linked to what we eat. Nutritionists and health professionals advise eating a low-fat diet rich in fruits and vegetables. These give us fiber, as well as a high intake of vitamins A, B, C, and E, and the minerals zinc and selenium. They help prevent cancer. Arthrosclerosis is another age-related disease that may be prevented by lifestyle changes. Dean, an Amish doctor in California, showed that a one-year program of strength management, exercise, no smoking, and a low-fat vegetarian diet may reverse the development of a coronary and arthrosclerosis.

What about the little adage about becoming senile? Many people think old age means losing their mental capacities. I sometimes think all of us do, regardless of what our ages are. However, I've found on my own behalf that I have gained incredible benefits from taking Ginkgo and lecithin, which has choline in it. Choline improves my memory tremendously. Some age-related declines in mental function can be prevented or even reversed with these types of supplements. Low cholate levels in the elderly can cause forgetfulness and possible depression. B vitamins are a nutrient required to produce new neurotransmitters. A deficiency in this vitamin may lead to peripheral neuropathy.

A deficiency in B12 can cause a disorder of the nervous system in which limbs tingle and feel numb, and can also cause delusions and mood disturbances. Many people think vitamin deficiencies always manifest immediately in poor mental and physical health. However, researchers have found that seemingly healthy elderly subjects can still exhibit low vitamin levels. In fact, an older individual can be lacking in certain vitamins for years without any outward signs of deficiency. If you are on medications of some nature from your doctor, you can rest assured that some of these medications are depleting your nutritional supplements. That's when you need them more than ever.

Regarding old age and losing teeth, you should be sure to see your dentist periodically. You can prevent most periodontal diseases. Store and replace your toothbrush frequently. Bathrooms are the most contaminated rooms in the house, so toothbrushes should not be stored there. Healthy people should replace their toothbrushes every few weeks. Those with a systemic or oral illness should replace them even more often. Good care for your gums and teeth is essential. I often brush my teeth with baking soda since it eliminates a lot of plaque. I also gargle with baking soda. It takes out much of the bacteria and is excellent for your gums and teeth. It is important to floss and get the debris out of your teeth.

The myths of aging are somewhat overstated. We grow old only because we want to grow old and we believe what people say. I have never believed in my entire life that I was going to grow old. I don't fight it, but I take steps to boost my energy and enjoy life. I'll have my intellect for as long as I live. My mind is sharper than it's ever been in my life because I've settled into the happiness of life, with all the ingredients that have been mentioned in this book.

It is also said that by the year 2025, we might know enough about how and why our bodies age to raise the average life expectancy to a hundred or beyond. It is definitely stated by many renowned scientists that there is no reason in the world why we should die before the age of 124. The genetic aspect of that really depends on us and how we take care of ourselves. Being healthy adds twenty or thirty years to our lives. Research into the cause of aging indicates that right now there's much we can do to add years to our lives and life to our years.

Essentially, there are two kinds of informed speculation: damage theories and programmed theories. Regardless of which theory is correct, proper nutrition, diets, and food supplements will help us. Our chances of a longer, healthier lifespan have never looked better. In the years that have passed, I have always been cognizant of my age. I would never share my age because I felt as though it was demeaning. I thought this was true for a medical treatment or on a job application. It's too late in life to do anything. This is all a myth. Without a doubt, never ever give up no matter what age you are. You can acquire anything and live longer because of it.

Free radicals are the carcinogens that cause a lot of the problems in our bodies. For longevity, we need to have the knowledge to fight free radicals. They are scavengers. Our antitoxins release the energy needed in our bodies without harmful side effects. When these cellular police are in too short of supply, byproducts of oxidation called free radicals escape. They start damaging neighboring protein cells. In the cell membranes, the nuclear material causes a buildup in cellular debris. Many people who are looking into longevity say, "Diet or die."

Another study has longevity scientists buzzing about weight rather than the caloric intake in human beings. They have said that thin people outlived heavier people by wide margins. What I remember most is that the heaviest people I have known in my life have died sooner and were more prone to the crippling diseases, such as diabetes and heart disease. Heavy people put too much strain on their hearts, and metabolically they need to get back into the realm of watching what they do in life. It's your prerogative and quest in life to be the best that you can possibly be.

A noted pharmacist has had many of his books out on the market for years. Earl Mindell has been researching nutrition for most of his life. In his book *Vitamin Bible*, he mentions the most important things he has discovered during his years of research: fiber, fish oils, garlic, ginger, lemongrass oil, lentils, pinto beans, lima beans, navy beans, monosaturated oils (like olive, peanut, and canola oil), niacin, oat bran, onion, pectin from apples and grapefruit, lactose sterols, polyunsaturated oils (like sunflower, corn, and safflower oil), and psyllium husks. He also mentions raw carrots, red peppers, bran, soybeans, vitamins C and E, and yogurt. These suggestions are coming from a man who has been researching these particular items for well over sixty years.

Some of the foods and nutrients that can lower your cholesterol naturally are: barley, carrots, chromium, corn bran, vegetables (like broccoli, cauliflower, and eggplant), evening primrose oil, and certain seeds. When I was working in the pharmacy, most of the people who were taking medications for their cholesterol never seemed to get it down. It just didn't matter what they took. It's a good diet that helps.

ANTI-AGING

I would like to discuss the power of anti-aging in a couple of different forms. One of them is looking at the life expectancy of the human being today. Scientific research seems to show that there is a gene in every person's body that never dies. There is something genetic they can't seem to explore or dissect all of its meaningfulness. One thing is for sure: Most scientists who have researched aging throughout the world have come up with many ideas about it. They believe some of the things that we are doing to live longer are related to modern medicines. Alternative medicines are also a factor. The life expectancy of a man today is 83.5 years old. Good health for a woman used to be a lot higher. Women are at a life expectancy of 85 years now. The men and women who live to be those ages may not be of the best health, but on average, they live to be those ages.

The scientific research on this subject is amazing to me because no one knows why an individual cannot live to be at least 125 years of age with a very fine quality of health. Doctors such as Deepak Chopra and Andrew Weil have gone to various parts of the world to study people who are 100 years and over (as old as 135-140 years of age) and what they do in order to live for such a long period of time. In America, we probably drink too much, eat too much, and maybe we don't drink the right type of water. Water is a very essential thing, and we will get into that a bit later.

How you view your life and how you choose to live it are both very important factors in life expectancy. Life expectancy has accelerated in such a dramatic way in the last fifteen to sixteen years. When I got out of the military in World War II, we were told that our life expectancy was forty-eight years of age. I was seventeen when I enlisted and got out when I was almost twenty. However, all of the men who had died in the service at that time during World War II had probably been taken into consideration. I was in the combat area in the South Pacific and naturally many people died at a very young age, and as time went by, it accelerated. In a period of fifteen years, the life expectancy number accelerated from forty-eight to fifty-six years of age. In another period of twenty-five years, it had accelerated all the way up to sixty-five and then to sixty-six years of age. The acceleration had continuously kept growing all the time.

Medical research has kept people alive longer, despite whether these people actually have a good quality of life. I would say that probably 50% of them, if they had used the natural form of medicating, would have extended their lives. I know that most medical doctors would thoroughly disagree with that. However, I think they are totally wrong because I have done decades of research and have personally tested what I've found. I have experienced many things in my life that I didn't like. I took the alternative and I am so happy that I did. I pal around with my sons. People keep asking me if I am their brother instead of their father. Remember, you have a good life ahead of you no matter what age you are! Keep hanging in there and discover the best thing that works for you. What may not work for one person may work well for another. Our body chemistry is different for all of us, so we have to find our own way.

The theories on aging are the hormone theory, the wear and tear theory, genetic control, the free radical theory, toxin elimination, caloric restriction, and the telomere theory. Less than twenty percent of Americans believe that we cannot do anything to delay the aging process. Even less believe we can turn back the clock. A good eighty percent of us regard anti-aging intervention to be either impossible or wishful thinking. I totally object to this thinking because I have a proven research calendar that shows what I have done over the years to prevent aging. I am often told I look about fifty-five! It's a compliment! There are theories behind preventing aging that really work.

The only theory that is proven to show an extended lifespan in mammals is caloric restriction of a nutrient-rich diet. It has been shown to work in rats and mice, and is now being studied in monkeys. While some people practice caloric restriction as a means of extending lifespan, its primary value is a model to explore how aging can be controlled. Research shows that by restricting the food intake of rats by 30%, they increase their lifespan by 70%. It's a proven fact that the less you eat, the longer you live.

In an article in *The New York Times* in September of 2003, studies found that teaching older people to relax or manage stress can result in a measured improvement in the ability of their immune system to protect them from infection. In one study, thirty-one people over the age of sixty were tested to gauge their defenses against shingles, which grows more common and debilitating with age. Some volunteers were then taught tai chi, which they did three times a week for fifteen weeks. Results showed that nine of the seventeen people in the tai chi group showed an increase with shingles antibiotics compared with three of the fourteen members of the control group. That is according to the study published in the *Journal of the Psychosomatic Medicine.*

Another study done by a researcher at the University of Bristol was published in the *Journal of Psychotherapy and Psychosomatics.* It involved forty-three people older than sixty-five, all of them caring for spouses with dementia. This is a high stress endeavor linked to increased risk of illness. Half the people providing care attended weekly stress management classes for two months. All forty-three subjects were given flu shots as a control group of similar ages and health whose members were not providing care. Half the stress-training group generated responses to the vaccination strong enough to form antibodies to protect them against the virus. Among the people providing care but receiving no stress training, only seven percent achieved that antibody level. Stress management group responses revealed that the control group only responded unless members were adequately protected against viruses. So in essence, stress plays a big factor in managing aging.

Some of the supplements that were found to have an effect on anti-aging with the research were coenzyme Q10, L-carnitine, lipoic acids, and natural human hormones like HGH, DHC, DHEA, estrogen, progesterone, melatonin pregnenolone (which happens to be a fruit), and adaptogenic herbs like ginseng, rhodoleia, amino acids, blue-green algae, antitoxins, vitamins, and minerals.

In this theory, there is a plan of action which contributes to anti-aging. Here is a list that will have great results. Gentle exercising, like tai chi and yoga, is great for your physical wellbeing. Massages and sleep are beneficial as well. Chiropractic care helps in many cases for people who are in a lot of pain. Organic natural foods, caloric restriction, and thirty percent less food intake are suggested. Avoid personal care products with toxic, synthetic, or proto-chemical ingredients. Don't use alkaline soap on your skin. It disturbs the acid mantle of protection. Be sure to have an adequate fluid intake. It appears that most people should be drinking six to eight glasses of pure water, rather than tap water, daily. The water from your household faucet has too many chemicals, such as chlorine and other toxic substances. I personally buy gallons of distilled water. Sometimes the minerals in spring water are not cleansing your body in a way that they should.

Eat fruits and vegetables high in antioxidants. All of the fruits on the market today are excellent. Try to buy organic, even if it is more expensive. If you can't buy organic, bring the fruit home and wash it thoroughly in pure water. Take whole food supplements rather than synthetic. Many vitamins and minerals are of a synthetic nature.

Avoid exposure to manmade chemicals in your food, water, and personal care items. If you must smoke or drink, find organic wine or tobacco. Try to avoid vaccines, including flu shots or flu mist. Scientific research is showing that flu shots are not something to do habitually, mainly because most of the viruses that you are trying to avoid are not the strands of microbial fighters that they are intended for. Basically, these shots are a no-no.

As far as emotional health is concerned, you should find fulfilling relationships with your family, spouse, or lover. Make love a part of your life. Love, in my opinion, is the greatest healer on earth. I've experienced it in my life and I intend to try to keep those who love me in my company as often as possible. It is always good to know that you are loved by someone, and it feels even better to be in a spiritual relationship.

Find your mission in life and discover a way to accomplish it. I have come to this realization maybe too late in life, but I doubt that. I am writing this book mainly because I want to help other people. This is what I enjoy in life. There was a time when I was looking for some form of reciprocity for helping people. I am totally amazed at the fact that when you are helping other people and expect something in return, it is an unfavorable situation and you do not get a meaningful reaction. When you do something for other people, you should never require or hope for something in return.

I remember being married to my children's mother and we would always invite people over for a barbeque or a party. Nine times out of ten, we didn't get much of a return or have people inviting us back to their homes. I finally came to the conclusion that reciprocity wasn't going to happen. However, I did realize that I invited those people over because I enjoyed their company. If they didn't want to invite me or have a return request sometime in the future, that was okay. You forgive people for those kinds of things. When you love, do it unconditionally.

There have been times in my life when I have not forgiven people for something that happened. To forgive them is the greatest health-bearing event you can do in your life. When you have hate in your mind and your spirituality, you'll never succeed with the happiness, health, and joy that you deserve. No matter how bad it may be and how long it has existed, you can always forgive. Avoid negative people and negative events. You don't have to be around people who you don't enjoy. If they are insulting, you can forgive them.

Be thankful for all your experiences. You can learn a lot from them. All of my experiences throughout life have been learning processes. I have just started realizing this in the last decade. There are many events that you never thought you would live through, but you did. You learn from those experiences. I did. Think about what helped you pull through those events. Keep learning and expand your horizons. Learning never stops, no matter where you are. It's never too late.

While we are on the subject of aging, here are a few little helpful hints on how to be happy. Yes, happy! When it comes to the pursuit of happiness, many people have it all wrong. They strive for a perfect life. If they can't boast of a solid stock portfolio, a loving mate, and model children, they sink into a rift. All of us have the power to make ourselves happy, even in the face of severe adversity.

There are a lot of secrets to acquiring happiness. Let's look at a few of them and maybe they'll help those of you who are not currently in that happy state. We all have personal goals—to succeed at work or a sport, or to maintain loving relationships. If these goals are not met, we are certain to feel dissatisfied. But we don't have to become depressed by it. There's really nothing wrong with dissatisfaction. It motivates us to improve our lives. The problem occurs when we become defeated by our dissatisfaction.

Sadly, this happens all too often, usually due to irrational and demanding beliefs. Some of the first steps to happiness can be taken by identifying the irrational "must" thinking. Change this to an attitude of "I prefer." For example, I'd like to have an intimate partner, but it may take a long time to find one. In the meantime, I can be at peace with my other relationships, or even alone. I have found it is difficult to feel alone. In the past decade, I have discovered that being alone can be informative about your thinking. It gives you an opportunity to work out your thoughts and think of the goals you want to set. On the other hand, demand is non-negotiable. It leaves you with very little emotional leeway. If you don't get what you want, you can become depressed or angry. An example of this is thinking you must have a steady partner, and that if you don't find him or her, it proves you are worthless. This thinking reflects the grandiosity of a child as he struggles to learn his limitations. Adults learn realism, but they revert to grandiose thinking in periods of stress.

If you can, try to develop a healthy attitude toward the reality of life. It's almost impossible to avoid. The trick is to learn to cope with obstacles without derailing your goals. You will have obstacles. They are necessary and are definitely going to happen. It's important to be willing to continue. Revise your goals if they are not working out. You must create other incentives to proceed with your life in a different manner.

Say that you decided to play the violin, only to discover that you have no aptitude for it. You can insist on playing your violin and drive yourself crazy because you are not as good as you demand yourself to be, or you can switch to the piano or another instrument that comes more naturally to you. There will always be alternatives.

An exception would be if you find a particular craft that is difficult to master, but still within your grasp. You may want to persevere until you are proficient in it. However, many people stick to unrealistic goals and look for more difficult alternatives. This is self-defeating. It is similar to Aesop's fable about the fox and the grapes. The fox wants the grapes, but can't reach them. When they prove unattainable, the fox derides them, saying they were probably sour anyway. I say it's better to accept disappointment about the grapes. Grab a banana instead and just move on. Don't stew about it. Just keep going!

AGE BUSTERS

There are a few big age busters to keep you feeling and looking young. Some of these things are necessary to understand your health and grasp the non-aging feeling. It also helps assuage your feelings of sadness and depression.

Number one: You should stretch every day. Stretch your muscles gradually and start increasing your flexibility. This will affect everything from posture to your golf game. It is great for back pain and tight muscles. To protect your back, do knee bends while lying on the floor on your back. Bend your knees up towards your chin and pull your chin forward to your knees. Do this three to four times every morning. Roll over onto your stomach and pull your hands and feet up into the air. Then roll on your stomach a little bit. Pull your legs together towards your chest and hold for three to five seconds.

Do twenty to thirty minutes of an aerobic exercise. This can be completed in many different forms. Personally, I run every single day except Sunday—my one day off. The amount of exercise is entirely up to you and how you feel. As I have mentioned before, I am a marathon runner and used to run 26.2 miles. I have discontinued that because I think it has affected my body in a negative way. I was very tired and sore for long periods of time. I now run anywhere from two to four miles a day. You pick your own pace. Walking, cycling, tennis, and swimming are all excellent aerobic exercises. If you seem to have a problem working out daily, add activity by getting off the train or bus and walking to your home or work, or park your car a good distance from your destination and walk the rest of the way. Don't worry if you think you have a time schedule. Just remember there is always time, whether you think it is there or not. The most important thing in your life is you! You deserve at least twenty minutes a day to do all of the above. It doesn't take that long.

Another thing you need to do is consume less fat. Everyone knows you should not eat a lot of fat. The amount of fat that you eat definitely affects the way you look and packs on the pounds. Reduce portions of meat, and when you do eat it, make sure it is lean. Buy lean cuts of meat and trim off visible fat. Bake or grill foods instead of frying them. When you do fry or sauté, use special oils, olive oil, extra virgin olive oil, canola oil, or peanut oil. Here are some more good food choices: fat-free salad dressings/mayonnaise, 1% skim milk or soy milk, and low-fat sour cream instead of butter. You should eat more green foods, cereals, vegetables, and fruits. I do so everyday single day. I eat some vegetables, but I don't eat as many as I should. Sometimes I take time out to juice my vegetables or fruits so I can get the amount that I need for good health. It is recommended to eat more vegetables and fruits, lean fish, and chicken. These natural foods contain more vitamins and minerals than processed foods. Make sure you stay away from processed foods. They immediately make you sluggish and lethargic.

Protect your skin. Try to stay out of the sun. Don't misunderstand—sunshine is excellent, but it has to be moderated. There have been many experiments done with different people on whether the exposure is good for you or not. The part of your body most exposed to the sun is your face, so it is suggested that you put on a baseball cap. Vitamin D comes with sunshine and that is one of the only ways you can get it without taking supplementations. Stay away from suntan spas—they will ruin your skin.

Stay away from over-the-counter medications, and when you do take them, read the labels to see how safe they are and what you may be allergic to. Never exceed the recommended dosage. When you buy over-the-counter products, they are just less than you normally would get in a prescription as far as dosage is concerned. Aspirin can lead to constipation and gastritis. Acetaminophen, which is Tylenol, can cause liver damage in alcohol users.

Avoid excess alcohol. I have a couple of drinks each night myself; it depends on your preference. Out of all the alcoholic beverages, I think the best come from Russia. Russians and other people who have lived for many years in certain parts of that country have always seemed to use vodka in their daily drinking regimen. That, too, should be used in moderation. Moderate amounts of alcohol are good for you—they relax you. Some alcohol even has medicinal purposes.

CANCER

Let's talk about some of the things that might prevent the dreaded disease that everyone seems to talk about: cancer. There are many scientifically proven foods which are often taken for granted that reduce your risk of getting cancer. Scientists and researchers claim that people never really talk about food supplements or foods that prevent cancer. I want to talk a little bit about some of these advantageous foods.

One of them is beans. This includes black beans, black-eyed peas, chick peas, garbanzos, fava beans, kidney beans, lentils, lima beans, split peas, pinto beans, white great northern beans, navy and white beans, and common baked beans. You can also look into soy beans which are getting a lot of attention due to their cancer-preventing capabilities. Possible therapeutic benefits include reducing bad blood cholesterol. Beans contain chemicals that inhibit cancer, control insulin, lower blood sugar and blood pressure, regulate functions of the colon, and prevent and cure constipation problems. Beans can help heal hemorrhoids and other problems.

How much should you consume of this so-called musical fruit? One cup of cooked dried beans every day is fine, but less is okay if you eat other cholesterol-depressive foods. Beans send your bad cholesterol (LDL) down. Beans also keep you regular and make your intestinal tract happy. They will prevent gastrointestinal troubles, like hemorrhoids and the possibility of bowel cancer.

Have you heard the folklore about beans boiled with garlic? Beans that are boiled with garlic are reputed to cure otherwise incurable coughs. Beans also are believed by some to relieve depression. That's an interesting concept, and most people like them. I certainly do, and I eat quite a few of them. You can't be around me too long after I eat them though because they do cause gas. That's obviously not too bad because it's better than getting sick.

Legumes are potent medicine for the cardiovascular system. When you eat dry beans, they are not entirely digested, so the undigested material lies around in the colon where some bacteria eat it for dinner. In the process, lots of chemicals are liberated and these chemicals act just like drugs that have beneficial effects, such as telling your liver to slow down its production of cholesterol. Your blood is reminded to speed up clearing out the LDL cholesterol. That's one reason why experts think that eating beans is good for your heart. A process called fermentation can also bring forth cancer-blocking materials. A primary therapeutic compound in dried beans is thought to be a very soluble fiber.

Dr. James Anderson at the University of Kentucky regularly prescribes dried beans. He says that a cup of cooked pinto or navy beans a day can help to lower blood cholesterol. He has documented that cholesterol levels sink by an average of 20%, even in middle-aged men with extremely high cholesterols. Over 260 mgs per deciliter can be lowered simply by eating beans. One man that he mentions who had a tremendously high cholesterol count went from 294 down to 190 by digesting beans. Beans sweep the bad cholesterol out of the blood and buck up the critical HDL cholesterol ratio. Moreover, legumes are regulators to insulin, so those who are diabetic might want to entertain the idea of putting beans into their daily diet.

It's a good thing to eat foods that have a good taste, and of course some of the ingredients added in the preparation of beans are the things that make them more palatable. It should be pointed out that less insulin stifles hunger, and a complicated mechanism may facilitate the excretion of sodium, thereby lowering blood pressure. Eating high-fiber foods like beans does lower blood pressure substantially, according to numerous studies. For example, vegetarians, matched for age and sex, had a diagnostic of 18% lower blood pressure than that of meat eaters. Even people with normal blood pressure have brought it down another 5-6% by bulking up their fiber intake.

Beans are also a cancer blocker. Legumes are concentrated carriers of protease inhibiters, which are enzymes that can counteract the activation of cancer causing-compounds in the intestines. In a series of tests, Dr. Walter Troll fed rats soy beans, and believes that other beans with protease inhibiters may have the same effects. He then exposed the rodents to a powerful X-ray known to cause breast cancer. Only 44% of the bean-eating animals developed an expected cancer, compared with the 74% that did not eat soy beans. Dr. Troll finds that protease inhibiters can turn off oncogenes, which are genetic carriers found in every normal cell. When they are activated, they may lead to cancer. Like beans, they may prevent the cell division, thwarting cancer, as well as the progression of the tumor. Beans are also rich in anti-cancerous compounds called lignans.

Although it's a subject that scientists can discuss at conferences with a straight face, beans are great for the colon. It is a proven fact that a greater output of large feces is a sign of good health. Scientists urge you to eat foods that increase the fecal output. They are convinced it is a way to alleviate symptoms or reduce your chances of colon or rectal cancer, diverticular diseases, hemorrhoids, and bowel irregularities. Beans decidedly give you a much larger and softer stool.

Dr. Sharon Flemings, the "dean of bean researchers" in the nutritional science department at the University of California, describes how she and her colleagues gave a group of young men a cup and a half of kidney beans every morning for about three weeks. The idea was to see how beans affected the functioning of their colon. Actually, the kidney beans were mashed into a paste, much like the refried beans we buy at the store, which many of the men ate on a tortilla topped with melted cheese. Dedicated bean lovers ate servings of at least three to six ounces a week. Others rarely touched them. The researchers concluded that beans are good for your colon. Beans decidedly increased fecal output and also appeared to stimulate colon bacteria to throw off volatile chemicals—short chain fatty acids that help lower blood cholesterol and blood pressure and possibly inhibit colon cancer. These fatty acids from the fermentation of food notably had soluble fiber in the colon and are being intensively scrutinized for their cancer-blocking potential.

For all practical matters, baked beans and other canned beans also count. Dr. James Anderson tested plain old canned pork and beans and found they lowered cholesterol an average of 12%. However, some Australian researchers recently noted that diabetics should avoid a particular canned food called legumes. They seem to create a high level of blood sugar. Looking at the cancer aspect, we should research and determine how many beans each of us can tolerate. Some people can handle much more than others, but this also takes all of the other heavy green vegetables and fruits into consideration. Broccoli, asparagus, and beets alone are fantastic for your health, helping the colon and preventing cancer. I should also mention that psyllium has worked in the prevention of breast cancer.

ALZHEIMER'S DISEASE

Alzheimer's relinquishes the brain's ability to think properly. There are many factors related to this, and scientific research has shown that gluten is one of those factors. Gluten is a product found in many grains. Of these grains, wheat is one of the most dominant. Wheat grains produce an enormous amount of gluten. Gluten seems to interfere with the neurotransmitters in the brain if we ingest too much of it. Yet some of it is good. We are exposed to gluten in many products on the market today. If you stop and look into all of the ingredients on the labels of products, I would say probably eight out of every ten that we pick up have some form of wheat involved. You should try to eliminate a lot of gluten from your diet. I have been told that I have an allergy to wheat, so I try very hard to limit my ingestion of wheat products.

I would like to mention some of the grains that are free of gluten. Gluten-free products include brown rice, long rice, long brown basmati rice, and things like buckwheat and millet. There are flours that you can use other than the whole grain of wheat: blue cornmeal, yellow cornmeal, millet flower, brown rice flour, soy, and soy whole. Some other gluten-free foods include black turtle beans, kidney beans, lentils, pinto beans, split peas, flax seeds, and sesame seeds. Some of the cereals that are free of gluten are corn flakes, boxed cold cereal, puffed millet, puffed rice, rice and shine, and soybean flakes. These will give you some indication of what you should look for when buying products on the market.

To give you some brain support, let me suggest a few items that have helped me considerably. I am very sharp and have great concentration. My brain has good circulation to keep the thoughts percolating. Let me give you a few ideas on the intellectual front. Your brain needs to devour mental challenges. Feed your mind with crossword puzzles, read books on philosophy, and challenge your mind with political debates. Physically, it needs nutrients. The brain's supply line is the bloodstream; therefore, keeping a steady circulation to the brain is essential for cognitive function. An active lifestyle and supplements that lower your risk of arteriosclerosis and blocked arteries hold the potential for preserving your brain's ability to work at full speed. A lifestyle that promotes heart and brain circulation includes consistent aerobic exercises and antioxidants.

Nutrients that I take are 800 IU of vitamin E and 3,000 to 4,000 mgs of vitamin C stretched throughout the day. These keep the plaque from building up and blocking arteries. Eat fruits and vegetables! I know you hear this day in and day out, but supplements of fruits and vegetables will restore the amount of nutrients that you need during the course of the day. Of course, smoking doesn't help brain function too well. Therefore, it needs to be eliminated.

I personally take as much as 180 mgs of Ginkgo a day. Around the world, the herb Ginkgo is taken to boost circulation and help forestall mental decline. Ginkgo is also an antioxidant used in China and Germany to alleviate dizziness, memory problems, ringing in the ears, and circulatory problems. For people with beginning stages of Alzheimer's, it has been found that Ginkgo can slightly slow the progress of this devastating disease. To further study the possible benefits of Ginkgo, the Office of Alternative Medicines and the National Institute on Aging are currently finishing up a study in Oregon's Health Science University of Portland and three dozen other universities around the country. The studies strongly indicate that Ginkgo helps to slow mental decline. In Germany, they already use it for those who have Alzheimer's.

SECTION 5
HEALTH CARE

OVERVIEW

Over the years, I've learned a lot about my health through research and going from doctor to doctor. It is important for you to know that you are totally responsible for your own health, regardless of whether or not you continue to keep a doctor for reliance. I personally think that trusting a doctor is the wrong approach. You should experiment and research. I learned so much from working in the pharmacy and understanding why most people take pills. It is the easy way out. People don't realize that there are alternative solutions. These alternatives all work; they just require time and effort.

For example, of the people who were coming into the pharmacy, I would say that about 95% of them did not exercise. I don't care what disease you have—you're never going to be on the road to success or healing unless you're exercising. When you age and suffer from illnesses, a cure might not work unless you are exercising. I think any practitioner who wants to tell you the truth is going to tell you exactly the same thing.

An important thing to remember is that intelligence is power.

Learning is power, learning is forgiveness, and finally, learning is healing. Educating yourself continuously throughout life will benefit you and keep you from the worry, stress, and other negative emotions that revolve around fear. I cannot emphasize enough that deep down in our mind, body, and soul, we are fearful because we do not know what the hereafter is.

PRESCRIPTIONS

Medical errors can be avoided easily. Each year, mistakes involving prescriptions and over-the-counter drugs cost the U.S. economy approximately twenty billion dollars in hospitalization expenses and kill almost 300,000 Americans a year. Here are some of the ways you can avoid bad medication, avoid taking the wrong drugs, avoid overdosing, and avoid drug allergies. Spend time communicating with your doctor before every doctor's appointment. Jot down, in the order of importance, all of the medical concerns or symptoms you have. If you suspect that a rash or any new symptom is drug-related, make it a priority to talk about. Most doctors have a limited amount of time to spend with their patients. Therefore, it is essential to start with the most urgent problem. If you ramble on about several other problems, the doctor may interrupt you, or you may get sidetracked and never get the help you need.

Occasionally, the physiological stress caused by seeing a doctor makes it hard to absorb everything the doctor says. In such cases, take along a tape recorder if you can. These are just simple things you can do. They may intimidate the doctor, but it is your responsibility to be informed. Be as diplomatic as possible when making a recording and let the doctor know that you are simply trying to avoid any confusion that may happen. I get confused because I get upset when I go to the doctor.

Before accepting any new prescriptions, provide your doctor with the following information: a complete list of the prescriptions you take (both over-the-counter and recreational), your vitamin intake, your alcohol and tobacco usage, and a list of what you take when remedying colds. Let the doctor know of any allergy or sensitivity you have to food or drugs. Women should let the doctor know if they are pregnant, or even if they think they are pregnant.

Questions for you to ask the doctor include: Are there any precautions or warnings that I should be aware of? Should I avoid certain foods, drugs, or vitamins while taking this medication? Is the drug intended to alleviate symptoms? Which ailment is the medicine for? Make sure that you receive explicit instructions. Never take a medication without knowing its purpose, and never stop taking the medication without consulting your doctor. Abruptly stopping medications can trigger irregular rhythms, and even convulsions and heart attacks.

Here's something that I think is extremely important. Try to avoid pharmacy mistakes. Some patients routinely ask their doctor to phone in their prescription to a pharmacy. Doing so can be a big mistake because drug names often sound alike. It's incredible how many blood pressure medications are out there. I don't know how a doctor decides on one or another because I think that every drug company makes one. Drug names often sound alike, especially when heard over the telephone at the noisy drug store. Ulcer medications, like Zantac for instance, can easily be confused with Xanax, an anti-anxiety pill.

Your doctor should provide you with a written prescription form. The form should be printed clearly in English and should include the drug's brand and generic names. It should include detailed instructions and should not contain abbreviations. When I worked at the pharmacy, I saw continuous abbreviations written on prescriptions. The pharmacists have to know exactly what the prescription says, or at least have an idea, in order to fill it. Do not accept sloppy handwriting. I think most doctors have the worst handwriting in America. I have yet to see a clear handwritten prescription. It's terrible. Every doctor should make a typed prescription instead of a handwritten one. You should be able to read it, and so should the pharmacist. Pharmacists might accept sloppy handwriting, but in a survey, more than half of the pharmacists acknowledged that a doctor's sloppy handwriting caused them to make a prescription error.

For instance, there was a situation in which a patient was supposed to get an anti-inflammatory drug. A patient was instead given Tolinase—a diabetic drug. She developed symptoms of paranoia, which is a serious condition. She had numerous amounts of problems with the drug and wound up in the hospital. If you can't read the prescription, odds are that the pharmacist will not be able to read it. Use one pharmacy for all of your family's prescriptions—that way you can be certain that the pharmacist is familiar with all of your medications. If possible, find a pharmacy that uses a computerized patient file system to track various medications. A good pharmacist can check on the computer right away to see if there are certain drugs that might have a bad interaction with others. Ask the pharmacist to check the computer for potential interactions and be prepared to wait. If you're impatient, you might get into trouble.

Your pharmacist should also check your new prescription for possible interactions with alcohol or over-the-counter medications. Sometimes these interactions can cause horrendous problems. An antibiotic, such as Tetracycline, can be rendered inactive by eating a single Tums tablet. Small quantities of alcohol can cause serious reactions in someone taking an antihistamine, tranquilizer, sedative, or pain reliever. There are certain antibiotics that you definitely cannot take with alcohol. They will put you into a catatonic state.

Like your doctor, the pharmacist should provide you with instructions on how to take a drug. I found that when working in the pharmacy, pharmacists can get so swamped at times, especially when everybody comes in at the same time. Everyone becomes impatient, including the pharmacist. Consequently, the pharmacist might not give you any information about drug interactions. It is up to you, but I'm making this imperative. If you know that the pharmacist hasn't got time to talk to you, you should come back some time when he does have the time. Sometimes the problem is failing to double-check your own prescriptions. Therefore, jot down the drug name and its dosage on a piece of paper. That way when you pick up your prescription, you can see that the label corresponds with the pill. If you suspect a mistake, call your doctor.

Also consider keeping a copy of a pill book. These are a physician's desk reference and there are many around. Be aware of a drug's side effects. Doctors are supposed to tell patients about possible side effects, but they don't always do that. Many doctors don't even know what the side effects are. A pharmacist is trained for that. I will validate the fact that pharmacists, in most instances, try to be as careful as possible, but they get overloaded with work. Prescription drugs can cause a variety of troublesome side effects, including sexual problems. I observed that many men came in taking certain drugs, especially high blood pressure medication, that definitely caused sexual problems. Their sex drive went down and they became impotent. For self-defense, research the side effects of any newly prescribed drug. Nine out of ten pharmacies now have sophisticated drug-dispensing software that screens for interactions.

I have even seen people who have become sensitive to a drug's color. Some people have a reaction to the coloring in a capsule and wind up in the hospital. That is not a big problem, but I have seen it happen over and over again. If you are sensitive to anything, be sure to consult your doctor. Again, stick to one pharmacy so you can always have a little brown bag of complaints that you can discuss with your pharmacist. That's like going to four or five different doctors, which many patients do. In this case, the doctors are not informed about all of the drugs you are taking, and problems are a certainty in that particular situation.

When you are combining prescription and non-prescription drugs, always check out the directions packet. In rare cases, non-steroidal anti-inflammatory drugs called NSAIDS, like ibuprofen, Motrin, naproxen, Aleve, and acetaminophen, can cause kidney damage. If you have kidney disease, you should definitely avoid a large dosage and not take these drugs for a long period of time. An acid blocker, such as Tagamet, interacts with diabetes medication. If you are taking a medication on a long-term basis, ask your doctor if over-the-counter drugs are going to interact with it.

Storing drugs incorrectly is a mistake a lot of people make. You've heard about drugs that are affected by humidity. Most of us store our medications in the bathroom, which is typically the hottest area of the home. All of your medications should be stored in a dry place, possibly in a cabinet in the kitchen. Try to store all prescriptions and over-the-counter drugs in a cool dry spot. If you have children in the house, make sure that the medications are up high so that they cannot reach them.

You should take the correct dosage of medication for your weight. Many people hang on to their unused pills thinking they will save a few bucks and a trip to the pharmacy if they get sick again. Yet even if you get the same symptoms again, taking old pills is dangerous. Your symptoms may stem from a different ailment. Therefore, if you have pills left over after taking a course of medication, you should discard them. If you insist on hanging on to the unused pills, at least call your doctor to get information about them. I have found that most prescription drugs have a six-month shelf life. Sometimes you are disobeying your doctor's orders when it comes to your prescriptions. An amazing amount of people simply don't follow prescription advice. Patients take more medication than what's prescribed. I observed in the pharmacy that those who took a lesser amount to start off with and built up to a larger amount had less side effects and complications.

As a nutritionist, I know there are some herbals that have interactions. I always inform my patients that there are five essential vitamins and herbs. They are A, B, C, E, and selenium. When taking these five, it's very rare that there would be any side effects or interactions, but even with vitamins it's suggested that you take just one for a while and add the others later.

Working in a pharmacy was quite an education! Throughout my life I've noticed that modern medicine appears to be only suppressing symptoms, not curing them. My beliefs were formed when working side by side with pharmacists for eleven years. The findings were a sight to behold. Modern medicine can do a good job. However, its treatment sometimes kills. For the most part, pharmacists do their jobs well. They fill prescriptions ordered by doctors. But because doctors' handwriting is terrible and sometimes impossible to read, they have difficulty filling some prescriptions. When a patient questions the script, the doctors are notified. Pharmacists do not like being questioned many times about the wrong drug being filled. I have seen pharmacists dismissed from their jobs because of errors in prescription filling. A pharmacist is only human and will make mistakes.

I was a nutritional counselor while I was employed by a pharmacist. Most of the time, I gave advice about trying alternatives. Some of the pharmacists objected strenuously, mainly because they, and most doctors, know absolutely nothing about the healing of nutrition. They act as though they do not want to know the value of supplements for prevention. Most interesting is that doctors and pharmacists do not intend to exert the time and energy to learn preventive medicine.

Every day in the pharmacy, I observed the filling of drugs for so many different patients. My most interesting observation was the strength and number of milligrams that were given. Patients large and small received the same dosage, regardless of their weight. Many small people could not handle the dosage prescribed. Most doctors, and by that I mean hundreds of them, all prescribed the same medicine dosage for the same ailment, and if it didn't work, they'd add another. I observed 95% of the patients taking drugs for a period of time. They gained weight, which was sometimes excessive. Working with scripts, I could always tell if the prescription was given by a psychiatrist since they would prescribe two or three different drugs. These put most patients in la-la land, and after a short period of time, the patient looked swollen and almost twice his original size. People sometimes put doctors on a pedestal, but I am amazed at what they do not know.

DOCTOR VISITS

I realize there might be a lot of controversy about the next subject I want to discuss. However, in my opinion, it is a fact. If you are an individual who is in the process of aging and you go to a new doctor, he/she wants your history before you even come in for a visit. Doctors will, as you are aware, ask you for your name, your date of birth, and whether or not you have insurance. They take all three matters into consideration for your visit. I bring this up only because if you are an individual who is age sixty-five or older, most doctors feel as though you're aging and there is not much more they can do for your health. They are so terribly wrong.

I have found from personal experience that when I tell the truth about my age during a physical exam, the doctor does not perform all of the necessary tests that are required for a complete physical. For example, many doctors only take blood pressure in one arm. When you're going in for a physical, make sure that they check both of your arms for blood pressure. Doctors will ask you what your symptoms are and how related they are to your health problems. It is best before you go into the doctor to not tell the truth about your age. If you are eighty years old, as I am, I give the doctor's nurse a birth date of at least twenty years less. The younger doctors think you are, the more attentive they are in giving you the necessary tests.

Here are some helpful hints that you may want to write down before you go in for your physical or visit. In your medical history, doctors are going to ask how your diet is, if you are taking any herbal or dietary supplements, if you get enough sleep, if you are physically active, and if you are experiencing sexual problems. You should also mention if you smoke, how much alcohol you drink, and whether you are having problems in your personal relationships. Try to keep the list to one page.

To save time, doctors try to take shortcuts during a physical. This can affect not only your diagnoses and treatment, but also your future health. Here are a few steps that are most commonly omitted. The one I just mentioned is your blood pressure, and the other one is your eyes. Most people visit an ophthalmologist or an optometrist, but if you don't see an eye specialist regularly and you are over the age of forty, your internist or family practitioner can certainly measure the pressure in your eyeballs. Test for certain things like cataracts and glaucoma. Also, have them check your hamstrings because few doctors test the muscles in your back and the thighs to identify potential back problems. You should ask the doctor to check out each leg to see if you have the right angles. The lymph nodes in the neck are typically checked, and your doctor should also check the groin area for swollen lymph nodes. Also, your doctor should check the pulse in your neck and groin.

Many doctors ignore the skin altogether, assuming that it should be done by a dermatologist. This is not true. Skin should be checked during a medical examination. If there is an oddity, the doctor should mention it and give you the necessary suggestions, especially for moles, the scalp, and the bottoms of your feet. If you have moles larger than one inch, or if your moles have gotten larger, darker, or have changed shape, you need to see a doctor.

Another place to check is the thyroid, a butterfly-shaped gland at the base of the neck. It is often missed during a checkup. Most doctors check women's breasts for suspicious forms, but few doctors show women how to perform monthly exams at home. It is helpful, when performing a self-examination, to move all eight fingers, minus the thumbs, and cover your entire breast area. For men, the testicles and the rectum should be looked at. I have been to a number of doctors over my years and very seldom do they test my testicles. When examining men over forty, most doctors perform a digital rectal exam and screen for prostate cancer. However, they often fail to perform a testicular exam. Beginning at age fifty, or even earlier if there is a family history of prostate cancer, testicles should be checked for PSA levels.

Routine laboratory tests should be done to test cholesterol, liver and kidney function, and blood glucose levels. Most of the time you get these particular tests done, there is one thing definitely missed by most doctors. I have to ask each time when I visit a medical doctor to get a test for C-reactive protein. An elevated level of this inflammation-maker can indicate heart disease risk. Elevated levels of the chemical homocysteine are associated with heart disease and stroke. The B vitamin folate, when taken at a daily dosage of 800 mcg, reduces homocysteine levels. Some people have a genetic condition that results in a lack of iron in the body and they might overload on this mineral through excess dietary intake. Elevated levels of a certain kind of protein increase the risk of blood clots. Low levels of magnesium can bring on fatigue, generalized pain, and muscle spasms. If you are deficient in zinc, an immune-strengthening mineral, you may be prone to frequent infections. All of these things should be examined by a doctor.

Through experience and working in the pharmacy, I noticed the prescription levels of people who were frequent visitors to the pharmacy. Many of these tests hadn't been done. The entire objective of this book is to inform you of the things that might be keeping you from achieving a healthy life. You could live to be 125 years of age according to scientific research.

Doctors are human beings. Therefore, they have certain days in which they feel better than others. There are many doctors who smoke and do not take into consideration that this is a hazard to your health. Then they tell you to stop smoking.

A doctor, like anyone else, is a human being and pays attention to those he has a good relationship with. Some doctors have to put up with many hardcore individuals. I'm sure that within their realm of tolerance, they have to do the best they can. However, I feel that you must be in control at all times when you go to a doctor. You must be in control of your life and know what you need and do not need. In my opinion, doctors load you up with unnecessary drugs. I have seen people come into the pharmacy who have been taking as many as twenty different medications! I don't know how they survive to take more. As time goes by, I've seen doctors change some of the prescriptions basically to do the same thing they think it's intended to do. Periodically, I would hear that a person who was taking all those drugs had died. I'm not saying that these doctors are intentionally destroying people, but I think there should be a limit to the amount of drugs that are dispensed.

There are all types of infections that go along with people who have been in the hospital. A friend of mine had a massive heart attack and then got a quadruple bypass. He lived only a year after his bypass because he had a strep infection. There was no antibiotic that could touch his infection. The bacterial infection that my friend endured was one that doctors did not know how to treat. They subsequently just continued to give him antibiotics of different magnitudes over and over again. Never once was it suggested to put lactobacillus into his body. The good flora had been totally eliminated from his body because of all of the antibiotics. Something so simplistic was never suggested to help save his life. He was only sixty-three years old when he died, but it was all because of what happened in the hospital.

Over 300,000 people a year die from an inappropriate drug that was given to them by their doctor. You've got to be in control when it comes to your health. I have personally been subjected to most of these things and want to make sure that I inform you of the other alternatives. If there was one alternative that was the master of them all where people never died, that would be the best solution. However, as we all know, life only lasts so long. We will endure if we take care of ourselves and avoid total dependence on a doctor to make us healthy. Hospitals do not want you to know that they are fighting for survival. There have been cutbacks from the federal government and healthcare plans have reduced their revenue extremes. Throughout the United States, hospitals are closing, merging, or implementing cost-cutting measures. It's not just hospitals that are at risk. Corner cutting also threatens the wellbeing of patients.

Here is what hospitals don't want you to know and won't tell you. They are discharging patients quicker in order to save money. They're cutting their nursing staffs. Even though doctors get most of the glory, nurses run the hospitals. They monitor your conditions, administer medications, and make sure your medical equipment is working properly. You have the right to inquire about the qualifications of anyone who is treating you.

Many doctors have a hard time with the English language. So you can misconstrue what they are saying if you are not familiar with their language. While working in the pharmacy, foreign doctors would call in prescriptions to be filled every day. We had a difficult time understanding what exactly the prescription was. This results in pharmacy errors. Broken English is no excuse for a sick person to have complications. Always ask what your prescription is for.

There are so many different ways in which you have to protect yourself. The hospitals reuse disposable equipment. Some equipment, such as a single-use dialysis catheter, is cleaned and reused. This raises concerns about infections and product failure. Although reusing equipment is not illegal, you are responsible to see that you do not get used equipment. Hospitals do not report inferior doctors, although the law mandates that incompetence or misconduct among physicians must be reported to the federal government. Sixty percent of hospitals have never filled out a single disciplinary report in the last decade. Part of the reason for this is that doctors and hospitals have the power to direct their patients to competing hospitals. Their incentive is to not make waves. Your best bet is to avoid potentially dangerous doctors. This is done by learning as much as you can about your condition and the medications used to treat it. The more you know, the better your ability to spot a bad apple.

Hospitals overwork residents and interns. Although current regulations cap the work hours of doctors in training, these limits may be routinely violated. If you are admitted to a teaching hospital, ask your resident or intern how many consecutive hours he or she has been working. These people lose concentration and lose concern, and this certainly starts interfering with your health. If you believe a hospital is doing anything that endangers patients, I recommend reporting it to your state regulatory organization. There are many ways that you can check this out. Watch out for PSA testing. Of the tests that doctors take, this blood sample test gives them an idea of what's going on and can help detect prostrate cancer. Look into it, folks, your life is in your hands! Do not, I repeat, do not, take total advice from your doctor.

KEEPING TRACK

When you are taking vitamins and minerals with medications, it's always good to keep track of your feelings. This includes how you're feeling, when you're feelings are not up to par anymore, and the like. With vitamin and mineral supplements, one suggestion that you may want to remember is that it takes time for them to work. Give a vitamin or supplement a good thirty to sixty days to show improvement. I have a multivitamin on the market called Ad-ditions. This product has Ginkgo in it. From my research with the E Commission in Germany on Ginkgo, they have tested it for over eighty years and have come to the scientific conclusion that you do not get the full effect of Ginkgo unless it's taken for a six-month period at 120 mgs a day. That's a long time for something to take effect. Its effects are numerous and almost miraculous at times.

This is somewhat the opposite of what medications from the medical field do. They suppress symptoms within a short period of time. There are so many pain medications out there and their accompanying side effects are unbelievable. The list of side effects often goes on for pages and pages. Some vitamins taken together offset the effects of another one. That's why it's so important to take them individually for a period of time. Taking vitamin B12 is good because it's so vital for memory and brain function. It's a vitamin everyone over fifty should definitely take. Unfortunately, B12 is combined with almost every other vitamin. It's destroyed during the digestive process. If you take B12 alone or with folic acid, you should wait at least one hour before you take your other vitamins.

DOCTOR VS. PHARMACIST

There is a difference of opinion. Someone goes to their practitioner who prescribes a blood pressure medication of so many milligrams to be taken a certain number of times per day. This patient goes to the pharmacy to fill the prescription. She wants to know, being that it's her first time taking this drug, about its side effects. This patient becomes alarmed when she hears all of the side effects from the pharmacist. The patient calls the doctor's office and tells him what the pharmacy told her. The doctor is angry. He does not want anyone else giving information to his patient. Next the pharmacy gets a call from that doctor. He is raising hell for counseling his patient. If you ask your doctor or pharmacist about alternative supplements, they cannot give you information. The knowledge for the patient is not there. They will tell you there is none and that alternative solutions are a downright lie. This is their only answer because most of them know nothing about vitamins or supplements. The patient is the victim.

If the patient will take time to research, he can learn how to combat most diseases in alternative ways. Of course, all options are open. You must take care of your own life. You shouldn't depend on anyone else but yourself. For example, Doctor A writes a prescription for Patient B. Patient B goes to the pharmacy to fill the prescription. Patient B asks the pharmacist what the drug is and what it contains. Patient B then asks for the pharmacist's thoughts about the drug. The pharmacist gives an explanation to Patient B. Then the patient calls the doctor's office to complain and relates the pharmacy's explanation of the drug's side effects. The doctor accuses the pharmacist of overriding his diagnosis.

The point here is that the doctor, the pharmacist, and Patient B all are confused, which happens very frequently. Now the patient has second thoughts about taking the medication prescribed. Just think—I am only speaking of one pharmacy causing so much concern. How many thousands of doctors and pharmacies and hospitals are being confronted with an error every two seconds? Research estimates 700,000 or more. You wonder why every day thousands of people are looking for alternatives, namely nutritional supplements and nutritional practitioners.

Working in a pharmacy taught me a great lesson. Always be cautious of prescribed medication and research any other alternatives. Recently I read an article stating that doctors are about ten percent correct in their practice. Maybe that's why the hospitals are packed with patients. Working in the pharmacy for eleven years, I have seen what drugs do to people who are really not that sick and have not been advised to take alternative steps. I worked at the pharmacy for the sole intent of observing how traditional allopathic medicine compares to alternative medicine, nutrition, vitamins, and therapeutic solutions that are obtainable, but rarely suggested by a medical doctor. That is the way the doctor is taught, and it isn't his fault. He is there only to treat the symptoms. If the problem is not cured, then he obviously will send you to therapy of some kind or he will cut it out.

Those are drastic measures. I have mentioned in previous chapters that I am not a purist. I don't necessarily think you have to be a purist. By that I mean that I periodically smoke cigars. I rarely ever eat any bad foods. I always pay attention to my health with the foods I eat, which include fruits, vegetables, and no fried foods. At the same time, I have a cocktail each evening, consisting of a bottle of beer of some kind. I have no shame in this whatsoever. For those who say that smoking and alcohol is bad for you, I have to disagree. I think they calm you down and ease some stress. The only way you can be harmed by these substances, especially smoking, is when you do them in excess. Anything that is done in excess is going to cause problems for you. You can eat foods of various natures, but if you pig out on heavy foods, you will become ill. There is no question about it— smoking cigarettes is very harmful for you. I don't advocate the fact that smoking a cigar once in a while is good for you, but if it is something you like, you can't just throw everything out the window.

Just to reiterate, I am not and have never been a purist, but I do love and want to be healthy, which takes work. I run, eat the proper foods, and take vitamins and supplements. I have experienced everything that you read in this book. Chemically, every one of us is designed a little differently. The good Lord, whatever he had in mind, made us all different. That is why we are human beings and visit all these doctors out there who are killing us with their medications. We must explore our own needs and discover how to fulfill those needs. We need education, and that is one of the reasons I am writing this book. I'm hoping and praying to God that it will help.

Many people have had successful experiences with the different nutrients and vitamins I have suggested. I have not been able to help everyone, but it was rewarding to help the ones I did. Hopefully those people have gotten off some of their medications and are living happier and healthier lives.

SECTION 6
TIDBITS

- Staying physically active may help reduce age-related macular degeneration.
- Docosahexaenoic acid (DHA) is an amino acid. It is found in fish and helps protect against Alzheimer's and other types of dementia.
- Smoking greatly increases the risk of cervical cancer.
- Restaurant meals have about 60% more calories than meals made at home.
- Don't smoke! Smoking lowers high-density lipoproteins (HDL) by an average of 5 mgs. Even secondhand smoke lowers it.
- Consider a drink a day. Alcohol can raise HDL, especially the larger, more beneficial particles.
- Limit your intake of starchy or sugary foods, as well as trans fat.
- Avoid some of the dietary supplements that claim to raise your HDL. HDL varies in size, and the larger the particle is, the more protective it is.
- Soda sales have declined slightly over the last few years, but Americans still drink 52 gallons per person on

average. Non-diet sodas and other sweetened beverages contribute to weight gain and the growing obesity epidemic. Certain sodas have about 140 to 150 calories, all from sugar. Is sugar in soda a particular problem? A twelve ounce can of soda contains the equivalent of about ten teaspoons of sugar.

- How does juice compare to soda? One-hundred percent fruit juices have about as many calories as sodas and other sweetened soft drinks, but they also contain vitamins, minerals, and phytochemicals, and if the whole fruit is used, you might also get fiber.

- Does soda cause heartburn? Research, including a study from Yale University, suggests that sodas can trigger gastric reflux and heartburn.

- Does soda harm your teeth? All sugary foods, including sodas, can cause tooth decay, especially if you continue to consume them frequently.

- Is soda bad for your bones? A Farmington Connecticut Osteoporosis study recently found an association between soda consumption and decreased bone density.

- Should you worry about artificial sweeteners in diet soda? The artificial sweeteners, typically aspartame, are somewhat safe according to the Food and Drug Administration, but can still cause some problems.

- Can soda help you lose weight? Though diet sodas contain no calories, it's unclear whether they actually help in weight loss, especially over a long-term period. A new review of studies from the United States and the United Kingdom found that food and drink sweetened with aspartame instead of sugar do help some people reduce calories and aid in weight loss.

- Natural healers and natural sodas found in health food stores and some markets may have a healthier image, but looks and advertising can be deceiving.
- Will drinking red wine make up for our being overweight and sedentary, or will it cause extra weight? There is some magic ingredient in red wine that prolongs life. It is an elixir. Hopes were raised recently by a study in *Nature*, a distinguished magazine. It found that the resveratrol found in wine is a molecule in the skin of red grapes. It has been found to prolong the life of some obese laboratory mice. A reduced-calorie diet, about 30% below normal, has been shown to lengthen life in monkeys and other creatures by activating certain genes. All in all, wine has some contributions to longevity.
- Anti-aging serums are a large industry in this country. Juan Ponce de León, a Spanish explorer who beat the bushes searching for the Fountain of Youth, is alive in all our hearts. Resveratrol may be what we are looking for. This is promising research. Apart from getting regular exercise, eating a healthy diet, and not smoking, there is no real anti-aging elixir, but wine seems to be one of the ingredients we can enjoy. Be sure you don't over indulge.
- Look into the consumption of prunes. To heighten the appeal to a younger generation and increase sales, the prune is sold dried. Dried prunes typically have a type of high sugar, firm flesh, small pits, and high acid contents. The most common variety is the California prune. Like other dried fruits, dried prunes have concentrated nutrients. A fourth-cup of about five dried prunes has 105

calories, 3 grams of fiber, and 300 mgs of potassium. This is almost as much as a small banana. It also contains copper borons, zinc, magnesium, and other nutrients. I eat prunes every single day, sometimes stewed and sometimes dried. Due to the combination of fiber and other nutrients, they make a great laxative.

- Pectin, a soluble fiber, helps lower blood cholesterol.
- There are practical prunes you can buy without the pits. They can be chopped or dried and added to cereals, yogurt, green dishes, stews, chili, or just about anything. They can be an added ingredient to help the taste of a certain dish. Soften dried prunes in red wine or Marsala and serve with a dollop of yogurt.
- Prune juice is rich in nutrients, but not in fiber unless it has pulp. It is relatively high in calories, around 180 per cup. Its potassium content is high. Prune juice is approved by the FDA, and it may help prevent hypertension and strokes. Prunes can help with many things, and you can even buy it in a gel form found in jams. It is available in whatever form you may want. I suggest you try prunes in your daily diet.
- If you are a man, taking an aspirin a day, even though it is really a pain reliever, may decrease the risk of prostate enlargement.
- Another thing you want to do is wash fruits and vegetables with water, not soap, detergents, or produce cleansers. The recent E. coli outbreak, caused by vegetables, has boosted the sales of special cleansers, but it is advised that you do not use them.
- Walking your dog, if that's what you wish to do, can help

you to stay fit and even help with weight loss.

- Make sure you get all the B vitamins that are available in many fruits and vegetables. Take supplements if needed. I recommend 100 mgs of all the B vitamins.

- To calculate your risk of heart disease, diabetes, osteoporoses, or other types of cancer, look at the website for the Harvard Center of Cancer Prevention.

- Working in the pharmacy for as many years as I did, I was very much opposed to taking statin drugs for cholesterol. But according to a recent study of 1.5 million U.S. veterans, although half of them didn't start taking the drugs until well after the age of seventy, the statin users lived an average of two years longer than non-users. The statin drugs may have some benefits which are just now coming to surface. The benefit of statin comes from its ability to lower cholesterol, but also from its anti-inflammatory properties.

- Pre-diabetics may have an increased risk of age-related mental decline. Be sure to look into the prevention of diabetes.

- The average American is eating nearly twice as much chicken today and 13% less beef as a result. We now eat as much chicken as beef. In 1980, we ate more than twice as much beef as chicken, but chicken generally contains less fat. Fried chicken is something that you should stay away from.

- Avoid highly processed foods. Beware of canned or prepackaged soups. Soy sauce, tamarind sauce, and most sauces used in Asian cooking are salt bombs. Watch out for canned vegetables and fruit juices, which are usually very salty. If you do buy canned vegetables or fruits, be sure to rinse them with water to eliminate the excessive salt. If your food is being made to order, ask the cook to abstain from adding salt. Reducing portion sizes will also cut back your sodium intake.

- Look for foods that have a lot of potassium. Potassium is excellent for your blood pressure along with other vital functions in your body. Americans consume too much sodium, and sodium seems to eliminate a lot of the potassium in our body. Potassium will help prevent and decrease the amount of hypertension you might have. The government recommends at least 4,700 mgs of potassium a day. That's what an anti-hypertension diet provides. Unfortunately, only half that amount of potassium is being consumed by Americans.

- Keep in mind that potassium is not great for all, including people who have impaired kidney function or have been taking certain medications. They need to limit their intake in order to prevent potentially dangerous arrhythmia.

- There are many simplistic treatments for headaches. One of them is placing gel packs around the neck, or running cold water on the head. Massaging the muscles in the neck, forehead, and temples may give some relief. One study found that an elastic headband with two small rubber disks positioned in the temple area helped relieve the pain of a headache.

- Relaxing can reduce muscle tension. Shift the tension away from the pain. When I first came out of the military, I had an enormous amount of headaches and found that acupuncture gave me the most relief.

- Biofeedback consists of hooking a person up to a device that feeds back readings on a psychological level, and may help with headache pain. Skin temperature, for instance, is related to contraction of the blood vessels. This may allow someone to have control over the pain. Preventing migraines might help you discover what triggers your migraines. It could be foods, too little sleep, or a beverage you're drinking. I found that when I discontinued drinking orange juice, especially in large quantities, my headaches completely disappeared. Other possible headache triggers are aged cheeses, caffeinated drinks, and alcoholic beverages, especially red wine. Sometimes chocolate with nuts is a big offender, as well as yogurt, sour cream, vegetable protein, and cured, processed meats.
- Hunger can bring on a migraine to some degree. Some people, if they don't eat small amounts of food regularly, seem to have intensified pain with a headache. Some herbs can relieve you from pain. Certain teas are excellent. They may have very little plant material in them.
- Botulism, a toxin, may paralyze the tissues, so stay away from it.
- Riboflavin, B2, and magnesium were shown to be helpful in several studies.
- People have found that hypnosis or acupuncture is good. There really isn't any good evidence but many people say these help.
- The American Academy of Sleep Medicine warns you to be careful when taking over-the-counter sleeping pills.

They are actually antihistamines and make most people drowsy. You can become dependent on them if you take too many.

- If you are trying to lose weight, it is especially important to exercise to protect your bones. It is best to exercise and cut down on calories. At the University of Medicine in St. Louis, there was a study that involved mostly overweight people who either dieted or exercised to lose weight. After a year, both groups lost considerable amounts of weight. Some lost eighteen to fifty pounds just by exercising and watching their calories.

- Don't expect a high-tech ventilation system to reduce pollutants from secondhand smoke.

- According to research, if you are a man who takes the hair growth drug Propecia, you should know that it increases your PS readings from forty to fifty percent. Be cautious of that product for hair growth.

- Small amounts of certain medical issues can cause problems with memory. Everyone you seem to talk to says that they forgot what they were supposed to be doing. Some people become a little alarmed by this. Medical science believes that one of the culprits that causes memory problems has to do with the endocrine system. Certain diseases are affecting hormone levels which can then lead to memory problems.

- Such things as a low thyroid function, which is a condition that affects one out of ten elderly people, and Cushing's disease, which affects the adrenal glands, are associated with the stress hormone cortisol that can cause damage to memory regions of the brain. Diabetics always seem to have a problem because diabetes affects the pancreas and may cause some memory problems. The liver and the kidneys may be accompanied by a little confusion and memory deficits. Cardiovascular problems and low blood oxygen levels are characteristics of heart failure, which can affect memory.

- High cholesterol levels can lead to plaque deposits in small vessels of the brain. They can reduce circulation, which in turn affects information processing and retrieval. As I've mentioned previously, I take anywhere from 120 to 240 mgs of Ginkgo biloba. It helps my memory level and improves the circulatory system along with information and processing retrieval.

- High blood pressure can cause blood vessels to deplete. This causes small bleeds in the brain that injure and kill brain cells.

- Lung conditions that negatively affect blood oxygen levels in the brain can cause memory problems. The brain can be impaired by a head injury.

- There are many people who claim that a tumor in the brain may cause memory problems, and of course anything that's going to interrupt the transmitters from other parts of your body to your brain definitely will affect your thought processes. Approximately 25-30% of Parkinson's patients develop dementia. Multiple sclerosis damages the myelin coating that protects nerve cells in the brain, and this can lead to memory problems. There are other common disorders of the brain that can impair memory or normal pressures. Lupus is another condition that can happen.

- Sleep disorders, like obstructive sleep apnea, are caused by a deficiency of niacin or vitamin B12. I have found through my research that vitamin B12 and niacin do wonders for improving your mental capacity and for healing disorders including meningitis, encephalitis, AIDS, and tuberculosis. Anything that's wrong with your body can affect your mental capacity.

- Alcohol abuse can cause memory loss. Sometimes when we overindulge, our memory is not as good as it should be. Or when we wake up the next day, we can't remember what we did the night before. Over-the-counter and prescription drugs can definitely affect your memory, especially drugs that include sleeping pills, pain killers, allergy medications, anti-anxiety medications, anti-depressants, and a certain class of recreational drugs such as marijuana, PCP, and angel dust. Drug interactions may also cause memory lapses and confusion. If you have or think you have memory problems, it's always good to consult your doctor. I'm sure most doctors, being human beings, know that everyone experiences some form of memory depletion at some time in their life, either young or old. However, it's critical to determine the cause and take the necessary steps to prevent memory loss.

- When speaking of supplements versus drugs, I prefer supplements. Ginkgo, lecithin, vitamin C, and vitamin E all help with increasing neurotransmitters in the brain. This will improve your concentration.

- Your immune system is the most important thing of all. One of the things that I recommended earlier for the immune system was echinacea, which builds up a good immune system.

- There are many ways to help yourself, but don't ever forget to exercise.

CONCLUSION

This book was written to aid those who suffer from many disorders which have never been diagnosed as anything of a serious nature. This book was not written to offend what the medical profession has provided for people with illnesses. Over the years that I have been researching and giving people advice about anti-aging, people have had many complaints about themselves. Again, I want to reiterate the fact that this book was written mainly to inform readers about all of the options that are available to them. Many people have gotten relief from supplements and vitamins.

I want to express my appreciation to those who have given me advice over the years. I have gathered all of my research though extensive reading and advice from medical doctors and health practitioners in the fields of nutrition, acupuncture, medicine. I have found that the medical profession usually never allows me to come into its schools and give lectures on the results of my research. Those who did accept me have found my advice to be very beneficial. My only regret over the years is that I was not able to reach out to enough people who need comfort and guidance about their health problems. There is a cause for every ailment, and all of the causes revolve around fear and stress. It has been my utmost desire to relate to my readers that, for whatever you have, you must first accept the fact of your illness. Get advice and determine its acceptability.

I must emphasize that you cannot depend on one practitioner to relieve you of your problems. It will be a constant search for as long as you live. Remember that the mind, body, and spirit are the elements of life, and when all other methods fail, I have always called upon God to assist me. He has been a tremendous help in overcoming my adversities.

To all the people who have given me advice over the last forty-five years, I extend my thanks and my gratitude to you. I am hoping and praying that this book will be a comfort to you.

Printed in the United States
138237LV00005B/3/P